The 15 Minute Back Pain and Neck Pain Management Program

Back Pain and Neck Pain Treatment and Relief
15 Minutes a Day No Surgery No Drugs

*Effective, Gentle, Quick and Lasting
Neck Pain and Back Pain Relief*

By John McArthur

Copyright

Published by **Natural Health Magazine**

www.naturalhealthmagazine.net

The information in this book is provided for educational and information purposes only. It is not intended to be used as medical advice or as a substitute for treatment by a doctor or healthcare provider.

The information and opinions contained in this publication are believed to be accurate based on the information available to the author. However, the contents have not been evaluated by the U.S. Food and Drug Administration and are not intended to diagnose, treat, cure or prevent disease.

The author and publisher are not responsible for the use, effectiveness or safety of any procedure or treatment mentioned in this book. The publisher is not responsible for errors and omissions.

Warning

All treatment of any medical condition (without exception) must always be done under supervision of a qualified medical professional. The fact that a substance is "natural" does not necessarily mean that it has no side effects or interaction with other medications.

Medical professionals are qualified and experienced to give advice on side effects and interactions of all types of medication.

Table Contents

There is a Lot of Pain in This World

Statistics tells us that back pain is the second leading cause for doctor visits in the United States, and lower back pain is the third most common reason for surgery.

It is estimated that 80% of Americans at some time during their lives have back pain - usually lower back pain. **Jerome F. McAndrews D.C., a chiropractor in Claremore, Oklahoma, and national spokesperson for the American Chiropractic Association** says: *"45% of those folks will have repeated "back attacks."* In other words 45% of people have chronic back pain.

Back pain is one of the most common medical complaints known; in fact it is the leading cause of disability for people under the age of 45. The worrying aspect is that most people are not even aware of the things that they do that are causing this enormous medical problem.

The good news is that for most people, back problems do tend to be an intermittent or temporary problem but it is also true that once you have suffered from a back problem, you become more prone to suffering from it again in the future.

Dr. Marc Darrow M.D. a board-certified physiatrist and

Medical Director of the Joint Rehabilitation and Sports Medical Center, in Los Angeles, California says*: "Back pain often appears to have a sudden onset without a known trauma or cause. Many patients state that they have never had back pain before and that it doesn't make any sense why they should have it now. The back has many tissues that slowly break down over time, eventually causing instability and pain. However, like a heart attack or stroke, back pain in the majority of cases does not happen unless precipitated by an acute or sudden injury."*

In Many Cases Surgery Might Not Be Necessary

The U.S. has the highest rate of back surgery in the world and evidence suggests that many of those operations are not necessary. More than 250,000 operations are performed each year. The immediate question is; how successful are these operations?

- The Cochrane Collaboration, an international network of health-science researchers, that review clinical trials, says: *"the scientific evidence for most [back surgical] procedures is unclear."*

- Studies have confirmed that whether or not a person undergoes back surgery, four years later the outcome is the same with or without surgery.

- **Dr. Hochschuler, M.D. an orthopedic surgeon in Plano, Texas**, a surgeon who has performed thousands of spine surgeries, says: *"If you're currently experiencing back pain, and you're thinking about having surgery to solve the problem, think again. If you can recover from back pain without surgery, you're much better off, surgery can have unforeseen complications, from infections to nerve damage."*

In summary then - surgery can fail, leaving you with more pain than you had before and most importantly, surgery is usually not necessary.

Alternative medicine offers a number of options which does not involve surgery of any kind.

Just like with any other ailment or condition, surgery should always be the last alternative.

Warning: You Have to See a Doctor When ...

Back and neck pain is a serious condition and it is very important to know when you have to see a doctor.

Dr. Stephen Hochschuler says: You should see a medical doctor immediately if you have intense pain that travels down your leg or radiates from your spine, sudden weakness in your leg or foot, or loss of control of your bowels or bladder. These symptoms are indications of a ruptured disk or other spinal problem and needs to be attended to urgently.

"Once your problem has been diagnosed by a medical doctor, there are many options for non-surgical professional care of back pain, including back specialty clinics, chiropractic, physical therapy, therapeutic massage, movement therapies such as the Alexander Technique, acupuncture (including techniques using electrical stimulation, such as electro acupuncture and Craig PENS acupuncture), gentle exercise therapies such as tai chi and qigong, and natural medical systems such as Traditional Chinese Medicine and Ayurvedic medicine."

You should also definitely seek medical attention for your back pain when:

- The pain lasts more than a week or so, and does not seem to be decreasing in severity;

- You have a back pain that is accompanied with an inability to properly control your bladder or bowels;

- You notice any other unusual additional symptoms that would not normally be associated with a muscle strain or ligament sprain.

Pamela Adams a chiropractor and yoga instructor in Larkspur, California says: *"Shop around and make sure that whoever you see is going to treat you comprehensively, looking at your lifestyle, your posture, your habits, how fit you are, how you relax, how you handle stress, and what your diet is like. Whether you go the allopathic or the alternative route to relieve back pain, see a professional who doesn't have a narrow focus."*

The Causes of Back and Neck Pain

For most people the most common causes of back pain is because of improper posture or symmetry and inactivity. One of the later chapters deals exclusively with the topic of posture and symmetry.

But it is not always easy to diagnose the specific causes of back pain; the back is a complex structure of bones, ligaments, tendons, fascia (covering of muscles and tissues), nerves, muscles, joints, fat, and skin making diagnosis of the cause of the pain very difficult.

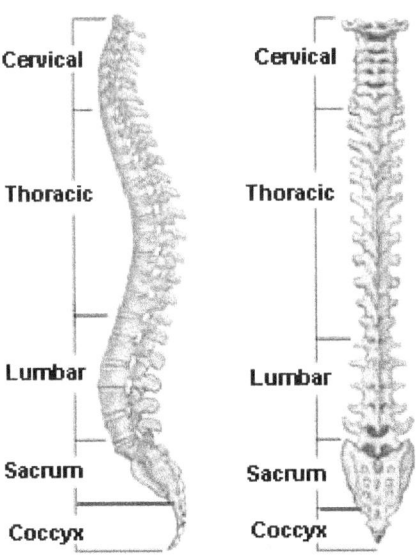

Dr. Darrow says it is important to remember that:

"Ligaments and tendons are basically avascular, meaning they have little or no blood supply to heal them when they are injured."

Your everyday habits at work and home are often closely related to back and neck pain. Think about it carefully; how do you sit at the desk where you work? Do you have to do heavy lifting? More and more of us spend hours every day sitting at a desk in front of a computer, but unfortunately the spine is not well designed for hours of physical inactivity. This inactivity, of sitting, could be just as damaging to your back as would be the lifting of a heavy object.

Similar in nature to sitting at a desk for long periods, is spending several hours a day behind the steering wheel of a car or truck.

Your lower back carries most of the weight of your upper body, which explains why so many times back pain occurs as a result of using incorrect lifting techniques, leading to strained back muscles and sprained ligaments.

Being overweight has proven to be another significant cause of back pain. The reason being that as your spine and lower back supports your body weight; there is simply too much weight for it to do so properly.

Other very common causes are sudden movement that jolts the back and damages a muscle, causing spasm, or buildup of stress in a particular part of your back.

There are also a number of specific medical conditions that cause back pain and we will consider these in the next section.

Acute or Chronic Pain

Back pain can be categorized as acute or chronic.

Acute pain comes on unexpected and quickly, sometimes immediately or within a few hours of an incident. Acute back pain is often the result of a sudden movement or something as simple as lifting a heavy object or an accident or fall.

Chronic back pain, on the other hand usually occurs after the acute stage and when the initial injury did not heal. For many people this means a lifetime of recurring or constant pain, which often comes from a simple injury like a low impact car accident or a fall.

Acute and chronic back pain are sometimes interrelated where the acute problem leads to a chronic one or, just as commonly, a chronic condition (which can be hidden for long periods of time) keep on causing "flare ups" - the acute symptoms.

Posture Plays a Major Role

Don't think that bad posture and symmetry only makes you look bad; the effects of bad posture are many, and can actually be really serious. For instance when you slouch, your head comes forward which also forces your shoulders forward. This leads to jaw pains, headaches, shoulder and back pains, it can affect your rib cage, which can damage your heart and lungs, and lead to gastrointestinal issues.

Dr. Hochschuler says: *"Most people with back pain have a problem with short, tight, rigid back muscles, and it can be relieved by improved posture while sitting, standing, and working; regular aerobic exercise; stretching; and exercises to strengthen the back muscles."*

Dr. Darrow says: *"The preamble to back pain is what I refer to as the de-conditioning or disuse syndrome. As we age, we typically become less active, spending less time in sports and physical activities. This process allows for muscles to atrophy. Also involved is the degeneration of connective tissue made of collagen, such as tendons, ligaments, and joint capsules. De-conditioning and degeneration can be traumatically induced or may continue slowly on its own via the natural aging of the body.*

This explains why the average age for back surgery is 42. Most patients around the age of 40 comment that they 'are falling apart.' In a sense, they are. "

In order to understand the causes of back pain, says **Dr. Mary Pullig Schatz, M.D., author of Back Care Basics:** *"It is important to understand the anatomy of the spine and its relationship to the rest of the body. The spine affects and is affected by every movement your body makes. The way you stand, the way you sit, the way you move, the way you pick up and carry objects all these things have the potential to help or hurt your back."*

Dr. Schatz says: The following are some of the factors that can be caused, or contributed to, by poor posture and movement, all of which can affect the proper functioning of the spinal column, inevitably leading to back pain,:

- foot, ankle, knee, hip, and pelvic alignment;

- poor muscle strength in the legs, thighs, buttocks, back, and abdominal wall;

- abdominal protrusion such as from a beer belly or pregnancy;

hip flexibility;

- the position of the pelvis, especially if it is tilted forward, back, or to either side;

- the position of the neck in relation to the shoulders;

- shoulder carriage and the mobility of the arms at the shoulder joints;

- the shape and flexibility of the lumbar (lower back), thoracic (upper back), and cervical (neck) spinal curves.

Doug Lewis, N.D., past Chair of the Physical Medicine Department of Bastyr University, in Kenmore, Washington says: *"One of the most common postural problems leading to back pain is a twist in the pelvis due to a leg-length discrepancy.*

This can be anatomical (the legs actually are different lengths) or it can be functional (the legs are different lengths because the pelvis is twisted). This can produce a lateral, or side to side, curvature of the spine (scoliosis), when it becomes pronounced enough. Anyone who has broken a leg automatically must assume there is a leg-length difference. Also, quite frequently, any injury to a leg during childhood or puberty, before the growth plates have fused, can cause a leg-length discrepancy because it doesn't allow normal growth of the leg."

Dr. Lewis goes on to say that muscles in the legs, buttocks, back, and abdomen, can become too contracted or too tight on one side or the other, which can also produce similar pelvis twists and leg-length discrepancies, as well as other postural deviations and spinal misalignments that can lead to extreme pain and physical impairment.

One of the most serious issues resulting from bad posture is spinal curvature. **The Chiropractic Resource Organization** says the following: *"The human spine has four natural curves that make up an "s" shape. When bad posture is practiced, the spine can experience pressure, slowly influencing the spine curves to change their positions. The spine is specifically designed to help absorb shock and keep you balanced, but as the spinal position changes, this ability becomes compromised."*

When the spinal curve is altered, subluxations may occur which is when a vertebrae becomes misaligned with the rest of the spine, compromising the overall integrity of the rest of the spinal column. This will eventually cause chronic health problems including stress and irritation of surrounding spinal nerves.

Subluxations can cause blood vessel constriction cutting off blood supply to the cells of the muscles, which can affect nutrient and oxygen supply raising your chances of clot formation and deep vein thrombosis.

Bone spurs (outcroppings that develop around the sides of bones) are another problem caused by bad posture and can cause a lot of pain if it rubs against other bones or nerves. In severe cases spinal bone spurs may require surgery.

Herniated discs very often occur in the lumbar region of the spine when the inner part (nucleus) of a disc pushes through the outer layer (annulus) of the disc. This can irritate a nerve in the spine, causing pain or numbness in your back, legs or arms. The soft discs provide a cushion between the vertebrae.

When your shoulders and back are hunched over it can cause pain and muscle tension in the upper back, on the other hand if you try to overcorrect your posture by pulling the shoulders backward too much it can cause you to tense your muscles and that could create pain and stiffness in your back, neck and shoulders.

Over time, shoulder pain and bad posture can lead to conditions that leave the shoulder permanently rounded (think hunchback) or contribute to joint degeneration in your spinal column.

Poor posture causes tension in the shoulder and neck muscles and joints and it will work its way up to the head, causing tension headaches.

A study by the **University of Maryland Medical Center** found that poor posture, while seated or standing, for long periods of time is a common trigger for tension headaches.

In Summary:

- Bad posture and slouching is not natural and if you are already a victim then there are stretches and exercises that you can do to counter the effects.

- Become aware of how you are holding your body as well as how you are breathing. When you breathe with the diaphragm, it changes your posture to expand your chest cavity causing the spine to become more erect, the shoulders are pushed back, and the head is pulled up. The key to gaining more energy is to assume more energetic postures. It sends a message to the subconscious that you are energized and ready to go. When you have low energy levels, you will probably notice that you tend to hold your body in a tight posture with your head slightly down and shoulders slouched. When you find yourself in this position, just start breathing with your diaphragm and pull your head up by imagining a cord affixed at the top of your head gently pulling your spine and neck straight and into alignment.

- Working at a desk and/or in front of a computer all day can force you to extend your neck forward and hunch your shoulders and you will wind up with back and neck pain. You should ask for ergonomically designed furniture at work, if you spend a lot of time on the phone, ask for a headset, so your neck muscles will not contract unevenly.

Here is a very quick and simple stretch that would help you relax those muscles in the back: *Grasp a pole or the edge of a desk to support you; squat partially so knees are bent; and shift your weight backward, as if you're trying to pull the pole or desk toward you. This stretch can be done a few times a day.*

Later on you will find entire chapters dedicated to stretches and exercises to help you correct posture and symmetry.

Physical Causes of Back Pain

Dr. Darrow says that back pain, with or without accompanying leg pain, can occur due to the following reasons:

- Stretch or tear injuries of muscles, tendons, ligaments, and joint capsules. Strains of the muscles in the lower back are by far the most common cause of back pain. A muscle strain is usually a rip or a tear in the muscle fibers that is caused by sudden force. Back sprain is caused by an overstretching of one or more of the ligaments in your back.

- Fractures, including spondylolysis (fracture of part of a vertebra that keeps vertebrae aligned) and spondylolisthesis (slipping of a vertebra backwards or forwards on another as a result of spondylolysis)

- Disc problems. Between each of the individual vertebrae is a small disc which is made up of a tough outer coating, and a gel-like central interior. These discs are designed to act as 'shock absorbers' between each of the vertebrae which in turn enables your spine to flex, bend and move in a controlled manner while not causing you any discomfort or pain (under normal circumstances).

    o Herniated discs or arthritic facet joint (joint between the vertebrae) that may impinge on a spinal nerve that courses down a leg

    o Degenerative joint or disc disease

- Injury, trauma, or arthritis of the joints between the vertebrae

- Pelvic or vertebral instability

- Inflammation of ligament, tendon (tendinitis), or muscle where it attaches to bone

- Vertebral subluxation (abnormal movement of a vertebra from its ideal anatomical position)

- Trigger or tender points (painful point or painful referral patterns from irritated muscle fibers or injured or lax ligaments)

- Tumors

- Fibromyalgia

- Local pain syndrome from inflammation of the fascia

- Muscle disease

- Spinal cord injuries

- Spasticity due to increased muscle tone with heightened deep tendon reflexes

- Scoliosis

- Osteoporosis fractures (typically in the thoracic spine, often causing kyphosis, or Dowager's hump)

Of course there are also back pain caused by rheumatic diseases, such as psoriatic and rheumatoid arthritis, ankylosing spondylitis, Lyme disease, lupus, and Reiter's syndrome.

Dr. Maoshing Ni, D.O.M.,Ph.D., L.Ac., President of Yo San University, in Marina del Rey, California says: *"Organic problems may contribute to back pain symptoms. For example, gallstones, kidney stones, infections, uterine fibroid tumors, and ovarian cysts can all result in severe back pain, because the nerves that go to these organs come from the spine."*

Sciatica: is described as a pain that not only affects the lower back, but also stretches down into the buttocks and legs. It results from irritation or overstimulation of a large nerve in the spinal column known as the sciatic nerve and can often accompany other less serious back problems like muscle strains and ligament sprains.

Spinal stenosis: This is pain associated with getting older as the spine becomes more restrictive because of factors such as arthritis.

Osteoporosis: This is an age related pain in which the

bones throughout the body get continually weaker due to reduced levels of calcium. Bones are gradually weakening and it is not uncommon to find osteoporosis has caused compression fractures of the vertebrae, particularly in older women.

Lumbar spine arthritis: Arthritis can attack any bone and joint in the body including the joints in the spine, making almost any kind of movement a very painful process.

Spondylolisthesis: is a condition in which a bone (vertebra) in the lower part of the spine slips out of the proper position onto the bone below it. When adjacent vertebrae in the spine become unstable because of a general degenerative condition in that area of the body, individual vertebrae can begin to shift their positions relative to one another. In this scenario, it is always possible that individual vertebrae will start grinding or rubbing against one another, and this will cause a great deal of back pain.

And if all of that was not enough here are a few very strange but real causes of back pain which very few doctors, let alone patients, will think of:

- **Psychosomatic** causes can also play a role as some people transfer their uncomfortable emotions into physical pain, which is easier for them to deal with.

- **Malocclusion** of the teeth-usually as a result of a dentist filling a tooth cavity or putting a crown on a tooth, especially while the back is out of alignment causes the back to become chronically misaligned, resulting in back pain.

Dr. Lewis says that he found a lot of back pain in smokers and believes it is related to the destruction of vitamin C in the body as a result of smoking. Vitamin C is necessary for the body to manufacture the collagen that makes up much of the connective tissue of the back. Defective collagen can result in lax ligaments and tendons or degenerative discs.

As for neck pain, the causes are similar to that of back pain. It can either be caused by incorrect posture, some strain in the neck, a degenerative disease or perhaps some type of injury to the neck such as in a whiplash.

Emotional Causes of Back Pain

The book Alternative Medicine: The Definitive Guide; Second Edition: Larry Trivieri, JR Editor, Introduced by Burton Goldberg describes a very interesting connection between psychological trauma and back pain. The case study is quoted below.

"Strongly held emotions, if unresolved, can eventually become fixated in the back and prevent the healing of back pain or successful recovery from back surgery.

Physicians at the San Francisco Spine Institute, in Oaly City, California, interviewed 86 patients (53 men, 33 women, with an average age of 41) who had undergone lower-back surgery. They found that if these patients had experienced three or more serious childhood psychological traumas, they had an 85% chance of not benefiting from back surgery.

Specifically, these traumas or risk factors included physical abuse from a primary caregiver, sexual abuse, alcohol or drug abuse in a parent or primary caregiver, abandonment, or emotional neglect and abuse (such as parents not being available for emotional support, overly criticizing or invalidating the child's emotional needs, or neglecting them). Even the existence of one risk factor reduced the likely success rate by 25%; when a patient had all five factors, the success rate was zero.

The researchers apparently failed to ask the critical question, namely, to what extent did the existence of these unresolved emotional traumas contribute to or create the back problem in the first place? But they urged doctors to assess "the pre-operative psychological status of a patient" before undertaking surgery. Metaphorically, the spine reflects how we hold ourselves in the world - self-image, if you like - and certainly children with serious abuse issues are likely to have a compromised self-image. Expressing this through the spine and back is, metaphorically again, logical."

Neck and Shoulder Pain

Important note: If you have sudden, acute neck pain, particularly after an accident or a fall, see a medical professional as quickly as possible for help.

Hope Gillerman, a certified instructor of the Alexander Technique (a type of posture and movement re-education) in New York City says that the origins of neck and shoulder pain (not caused by an injury/accident) is usually by neck muscles tightening, lifted shoulders, and the wrong breathing (gasped, really) from high in your chest. This is what is called a "startle response".

The pace and demands of our modern society get us stuck in a constant state of stress which causes this "startled" response. And the problem doesn't stop there. Because the breathing is shallow, those tight, painful neck and shoulder muscles are deprived of oxygen, which causes even more tension and pain.

There's no reason, however, for you to stay stuck in startle mode, Gillerman says.

Movement therapies, such as the Alexander Technique, Hellerwork and Feldenkrais are very effective to help relief neck and shoulder pain. There is also more detail about those techniques later in this book.

Chiropractic treatments that adjust the vertebrae can also effectively relieve chronic neck and shoulder pain, says **Michael D. Pedigo, D.C., a chiropractor in San Leandro, California**.

Other alternative therapies that may help are acupuncture, massage therapy, and craniosacral therapy (an osteopathic technique that focuses on the muscles and bones in the head and neck area).

Breathing: Complete the Exhale

Gillerman says: *"The best way to use breathing to reduce pain in your neck and shoulders-in fact, anywhere in your body-is to focus on completing the exhalation rather than assisting the inhalation."*

Extending the exhale is natural. It's exactly what we do when we speak. In fact, a simple way to complete the exhale is by speaking very quietly and counting to 10 over and over until you have no more air left, then letting air come back in through either your mouth or your nose."

Be careful not to stress, fully push the air out as your exhale is nearing completion. Just count until the exhale is naturally finished, without squeezing or forcing air out of your lungs. Repeat five times in a row.

You can do this exercise as frequently as you like, especially any time your neck and shoulders feel tight".

Breathing: Let Go of Tension

Gillerman says the next step is to discover the exact location of the tension.

"You can't let go of tense muscles unless you feel the tension," she says.

Place one palm on the back of your neck. Tighten your neck muscles by jutting your chin forward.

Hold for 2 seconds, then return your head and chin to their normal position while focusing on the muscles you've just tightened, and lift the back of your head off your shoulders.

Put your attention on the tight area (neck muscles) and then say to yourself, 'I allow my neck to be soft and free.' The muscles there will immediately become less tense.

Repeat this process each morning and at night before you go to bed."

Relax On Your Back

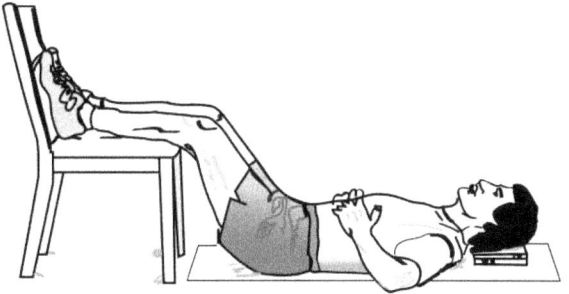

Gillerman says: *"You'd think that lying flat on your back would be a great way to relax your tense neck and shoulders. When you lie flat on your back, your neck arches, your chin lifts, and your forehead drops back, which is a constricting position for the neck and shoulder muscles.*

Instead, lie on a well-carpeted floor, a rug, or an exercise mat, and put between 1 and 3 inches of support under your head (your skull, not your neck). That's about the thickness of one or two paperback books.

This places the chin and the forehead in line-in other words, the chin is not higher than the forehead, which relaxes the neck and shoulders.

Bend your knees by resting your calves on the seat of a chair or a couch, or just put a couple of pillows under each knee.

Then bend your elbows and place your hands on your ribs. (Lying with your hands by your sides rolls your shoulders forward, making it harder to let go of shoulder tension.) As a variation, if you have a lot of tension between your shoulder blades, lie with your arms crossed over your chest.

This is a great position for letting go of tension and relieving pain."

Lying like this for 10 to 15 minutes a day (after work is a great time), focus on your tight neck and shoulder muscles and use affirmations such as *"I allow my neck to be soft and free; I allow my shoulders and chest to be soft and wide."*

Shake Off the Tension

Shoulder shrugs are a great way to relief neck and shoulder pain. Just lift your shoulders easily and let them flop down a couple of times. Don't push them down let them drop freely. Do these whenever you've been sitting for a long time.

Take a Short Break Every Hour

If you are working at a desk and/or in front of a computer, you should stand at least once every hour. Take a sort walk.

Even when you are sitting down, try to change your

position and shift your body weight whenever possible, because it is the inactivity that can adversely affect your neck and shoulders and cause pain.

In the later chapters you will find a number of excellent therapeutic stretches and exercises that will be of great help to relief your neck and shoulder pain.

Quick Pain Relief Techniques

Emergencies

In scenarios where you get injured in an accident or any other sudden event and if you suspect any fractures or serious injury seek help to get you to an emergency facility for X-rays or a complete examination.

If you are confident that you have not sustained any serious injury, move carefully to the nearest soft floor surface and lie down.

Try to relieve the muscular tension by doing some of the very gentle stretches described later on in this book, it will help to relax the muscles, decompress the spine and release any pressure on the nerves. But make sure you don't increase the pain or make it worse.

Next employ the heat and ice treatment described below.

Heat and Ice Treatment

The application of either heat or ice may help to alleviate the severity of back and neck pain. After assessing the problem, decide which of the two alternatives seems most appropriate. Keep in mind the fact that what is good for one person will not necessarily be most appropriate for another.

You might need to test both alternatives; however it is advised to use cold therapy first because the application of heat could exacerbate any swelling or inflammation, whereas the application of ice tends to be friendlier.

Here are some guidelines to help you decide when to use heat and when to use ice.

Use ICE when:

You have a back muscle injury and there is any swelling or inflammation.

Ice narrows the blood vessels that will limit internal bleeding and swelling.

Wrap the ice in a cloth or towel to prevent discomfort or 'ice burn' and apply for 10 to 15 minutes at a time. After application, allow your skin temperature to return to normal before repeating the process as many times as necessary.

Do not introduce <u>heat</u> for at least 48 hours (and even longer if there is swelling present).

If your back pain is caused by excess or unaccustomed physical activity or exercise, then the application of an ice pack may be the most appropriate solution.

Dr. David Bresler, Ph.D., L.Ac. of Los Angeles, California says: *"Ice is probably the most effective method for treating back pain, particularly acute cases.*

This is especially true when there is swelling, heat, or redness surrounding the painful area. Ice allows the blood to reabsorb the fluids and chemicals that surround the injured area and is particularly effective during the first few days of treatment. A standard treatment for back pain is to apply ice for ten minutes, then a hot water bottle (not an electric heating pad) for five minutes, then reapply ice, heat, and ice once more for the same amount of time. This can be repeated as often as needed throughout the day.

However, if the swelling and pain continues consult a doctor immediately."

Use HEAT when:

If there is no swelling use heat to reduce the pain

Heat works best for chronic pain.

Applying heat to a muscle increases its flexibility and elasticity and will encourage movement in your muscles.

Heat increases blood flow and skin temperature, moist heat is best, try using a hot towel for 15 to 20 minutes at a time.

You can repeat this process as many times as necessary for three or four days, but if the problem persists its time to seek appropriate medical advice.

No Drug Pain Relief

Obviously you can use over the counter or prescription anti-inflammatory medications for pain relief but you must keep in mind that they could have nasty side effects, including digestive upset.

The good news is that there is a natural medicine called MSM (methylsulfonylmethane) that may work just as well.

MSM has proved to be very effective for treating chronic back pain, says **Dr. Stanley W. Jacob, M.D., professor of surgery at Oregon Health Sciences University in Portland.**

"I have seen several hundred patients for back pain secondary to other problems, such as arthritis, disk degeneration, and accidents. For such pain-related conditions, MSM is usually beneficial. In fact, there may be no pharmaceutical therapy that is

better."

Dr. Jacob recommends taking up to 8 grams of MSM a day in divided doses with meals.

Because the supplement may cause loose stools, start with 2 grams daily and increase by 2 grams every 7 days, if necessary, until you reach 8 grams. (Increase the dosage only if the lower dosage does not help.) This should help you avoid bowel problems, says Dr. Jacob.

Important Note: If you're being treated with a blood-thinning drug, take MSM only with your doctor's approval and supervision, since it may thin the blood slightly.

Otherwise, says Dr. Jacob, MSM is a safe supplement with no serious side effects.

Massage Might Help Quickly

Many people find that enjoying a good massage will help to alleviate their back pain problems.

A new study demonstrates that massage is a superior treatment option to both acupuncture and self-care.

Experts agree that often the best way to manage chronic

back pain is to use several therapies at once, and therapeutic massage may be an important part of the package.

Dr. Daniel C. Cherkin, PhD says: *"There is some scientific evidence that massage may be useful for people with chronic back pain. Therefore, it's certainly something that one with chronic back pain should consider trying."*

Dr. Michael Hirt, MD, medical director of the Center for Integrative Medicine at the Encino-Tarzana Regional Medical Center in Los Angeles says: *"Millions of people use massage therapeutically and there's not a lot of hard evidence that it works. This is one of the few well-conducted studies that shows there's some significant benefit, and the benefit might be higher than for some other alternative therapies that we consider to be effective for pain, like acupuncture. ... Three out of four people who had massage therapy in this study showed benefit, and that's legions above the kind of benefits we see with physical therapy or medications."*

13 Non-Surgical Treatment Options

For any treatment to be effective it is critical to know what the root cause of the problem is.

Dr. Doug Lewis, N.D., past Chair of the Physical Medicine Department of Bastyr University, in Kenmore, Washington says in many cases the wrong approach to the treatment of back pain is followed by physicians: *"The symptoms of back pain are treated without regard for their underlying causes. The site of the pain is rarely the site of the dysfunction. You may make the pain subside, but you're not correcting the dysfunction that caused the pain in the first place. If you leave the pain alone and treat the cause, then you have the pain as a monitor for whether or not your therapy is working."*

Dr. Lewis gives the following account of an experience he had with a lower back pain patient: *"I treated her for the seeming indications of her pain, and she'd go away and feel great for two or three days, and then by the following week she'd be back in, with exactly the same complaint, exactly the same intensity. We did this several times, with the same result, until finally I said to her, 'I think you should see a gynecologist.' She had an exam and discovered a grapefruit-sized cyst on her right ovary, which was removed, and immediately all of her back pain went away."*

On the other hand Dr. Lewis says he also found that the reverse can also occur: *"If there's a chronic dysfunction in the musculoskeletal part of the system, it can negatively influence what happens with the organs. Quite often when I have patients with severe or even mild dysmenorrhea (pain associated with menstruation), I will treat the lower back and that will relieve the dysmenorrhea."*

People with back pain can choose from any number of alternative approaches, including all the various physical manipulation techniques and movement awareness therapies, mind/body medicine, energy medicine, acupuncture, and naturopathy.

Ideally, an alternative practitioner will help the patient explore all the treatment possibilities available and encourage him or her to take an active role in the treatment process.

- Because many cases of back pain are muscular in origin, the pain usually occurs as a result of the way a person uses, or misuses, his or her body. Most back pain can be avoided by taking the simple preventative step of staying in good physical condition.

- Physical manipulation techniques aim to move the various

parts of the back-muscles, connective tissues, and vertebrae-into proper functional alignment and can often correct serious problems relating to stress and physical pain. Options include chiropractic, osteopathic, and bodywork therapies.

- As well as being an excellent way to keep the body limber and in shape, yoga breathing exercises and postures, Tai Chi, or Qigong have the potential to reduce much of the tension and stress that can contribute to back and neck pain.

- Prolotherapy, also known as regenerative therapy or sclerotherapy, is a technique that can dramatically reduce or eliminate back pain. More about that later.

- Mind/body techniques such as guided imagery and biofeedback may be helpful for relieving back pain.

- Energy medicine techniques, such as ultrasound, the TENS unit, micro-current stimulators, soft lasers, and infrared lights, have been used successfully to treat back pain.

- Many studies have shown the effectiveness of acupuncture or acupressure for treating back pain.

- One very simple yet effective and completely natural way of getting rid of your back pain is to stay in bed for a couple of days. Give it a rest.

If you suffer chronic back pain or are at high risk for back pain you should consider making whatever lifestyle changes are necessary such as working on your symmetry and posture and doing strengthening exercises.

The moral of the story is therefore that there are so many different factors that contribute to back pain; it is of the utmost importance to know what causes the problem in order to choose the best treatment. For instance your problem could be as simple as noticing and changing the way you're sitting.

Always remember that in most cases back pain can be relieved without having to go through surgery.

Dr. Darrow says: *"Each medical discipline seems to find the diagnosis of back pain within the standards of what it is taught. Often, a patient will be diagnosed with several different causes of pain by different practitioners. This is very confusing to the patient, who doesn't know whom to believe."*

Dr. Darrow's views are supported by **Dr. David Bresler, Ph.D., of Los Angeles, California, former Director of the U.C.L.A. Pain Center:** *"When you're dealing with back pain, the type of therapy someone gets often depends on the type of doctor he or she goes* to see. When you see an orthopedist, you'll get physical therapy and cortisone, maybe even surgery. If you see a physiatrist, you'll get exercises and maybe some physical therapy. If you see a chiropractor, you'll get adjusted, and if you see an acupuncturist, you'll get needled. It's a rather arbitrary way to determine what's best for a patient."

Dr. Bresler tailors his approach to the specific needs of each patient and, if it seems appropriate, he will refer the person to someone else.

Dr. Darrow says that his patients rarely end up "under the knife." *"About 90% of my back pain patients have nothing more than sprained or lax ligaments, or a strain of a muscle where it attaches to bone. Surgery simply cannot help them. My office is filled with patients who come to us after failed surgeries."*

Prevention is Better than Cure

Did you know that your posture, back health, and how you move can actually be an indicator of how old your body is? **Joseph Pilates** said: *"The age of your body is in direct relation to the age of your spine."*

So, if you have a healthy back you will not only feel younger but look younger too!

What a great concept. Keep your spine healthy and you will be healthy!

Your back health should start with stretches and exercises that can help you improve the age of your spine.

In the majority of people back pain is caused by some sort of muscular problem which usually occurs as a result of the way a person uses, or misuses, his or her body. The way people sit, stand, and walk puts strain on the back, pushing and pulling the spine out of alignment and causing weakness, spasms, and sprains in tendons, ligaments, and muscles.

The end result of these bad habits is pain in the back and/or neck or pain referred through the nervous system to other parts of the body i.e. the legs, shoulder or arms.

Getting and staying in good physical condition can avoid back pain. Research has shown that exercise can also benefit the treatment of low back pain, especially exercise programs that maintain and strengthen the lower back and spine. These include aerobic exercises, stretches, and strengthening exercises such as sit-ups. These both help to stabilize the pelvis and progressively increase the free range of movement of the back.

Later on in the book you will find chapters that deal

extensively with various stretching and exercise routines which you can follow.

Proper movement is another key to a strong and healthy back which can prevent pain. Many people tend to over-tighten their muscles in the arms, legs, neck, and back when they walk. This can be can be corrected if they can learn how to use the body more efficiently and how to rectify symmetry and postures through an ongoing process of exercise and self-awareness.

Lose Weight it WILL Ease the Load on Your Back

Weight loss and maintaining a healthy weight level is another excellent preventative measure.

As with any medical condition, rather than waiting for a back and/or neck pain problem to develop, it makes far more sense to take steps before you ever suffer the discomfort of back and/or neck pain to take steps to ensure that you never do so.

If you want to know what your body is going through just take a bag and fill it to the weight equivalent to what you are overweight, then go for a 30 minute walk while carrying it. You will soon physically experience and realize what you are doing to your body by being overweight.

If you are overweight or obese, you are at a significantly higher risk of suffering back problems and therefore you should begin to shed the extra weight as soon as possible.

Of course, this will not only benefit your back, your general health will increase significantly as you shed the extra bulk that is undoubtedly putting a strain on your body and spine.

Prevention is always better than having to find a cure and prevention is to a very large extent in your own hands. So you have to make the choice.

A Good Rest Can Do Wonders

It might not be a surprise but in case you did not know; rest is one of the most effective back pain treatment options you can get. Rest has proven to be effective even in serious cases such as a slipped disc. Rest should almost always be your first treatment option.

With the bed rest your doctor might also prescribe some anti-inflammatory drugs or if you don't want to take those you can ask your doctor to prescribe MSM as noted before.

Although bed rest is a great way of reducing the severity of the pain, be aware that you could have too much of a good thing.

You should not stay in bed for more than two or three days as it weakens the muscles if they don't move for long periods of time.

Does the type of bed make any difference? Your choice of bed is an absolutely critical factor in how much back pain relief you will get from bed rest. But don't worry you don't necessarily need an orthopedic bed or mattress. In fact, according to research in the UK, the majority of orthopedic mattresses are too hard, and as a result, only 6% of experts would recommend an orthopedic mattress to back pain sufferers.

You are looking for a mattress that is firm and supportive, as opposed to being hard. Everyone who suffers from back pain has a slightly different problem and therefore there is not one ideal sleeping solution that covers every back pain sufferer. You must be willing to do a little research when you buy your next bed. That bed could be the difference between your continuing to suffer and solving your problems.

Also don't forget that the right type of pillow might do wonders for your neck, shoulders and upper back. These days there are very nice and comfortable therapeutic full body and other types of pillows that can be very helpful. It might be all you need.

Also see later in the book about posture when you sleep in order to work out what would be your best sleeping position. In some cases its best to be on your back while in other it's best to be on your stomach and in some cases on your side.

Magnet Therapy

Many people believe that magnet therapy is quackery and if you talk to conventional doctors most of them will tell you so. But don't believe that, there is lots of scientific proof that magnets can be in some cases a very effective back and neck pain treatment option.

Julian Whitaker, M.D. **director of the Whitaker Wellness Institute in Newport Beach, California** used to have lower-back pain and he says: *"I used to get up in the morning, let my legs flop out of bed, and then limp around for quite a while. Now, I don't notice any back pain."*

He says this is what he did: *"I used a corset with magnets inserted in it. A magnetic field may help relieve pain by increasing blood flow to the injured area or by altering the transmission of pain in nerve fibers. I wear my corset under my clothes, I sleep in it-I wear it everywhere except for the shower."*

He recommends using magnets of 3,000 to 4,000 gauss,

although magnets with strengths as low as 500 gauss have been shown to relieve back pain.

Note: Gauss is a measure of a magnet's strength; a refrigerator magnet is a little less than 300 gauss. Never try to use refrigerator magnets.

There are lots of theories as to how magnets work to relief pain and as far as I could see the jury is still out. Despite the fact that we don't understand exactly how magnets really work when it comes to pain relief it has been proven beyond doubt that they do work and are safe to use if used correctly.

Magnets are not a means on their own to 'fix' a bad back but they somehow help by assisting to regain the body's natural balance, especially after an incident or accident when there's inflammation and swelling present.

Magnets (quality and correct magnets), come in a range of shapes, sizes, styles and applications. You can get them in mattress overlays, you can wear them around your waist, your neck, wrist or pretty much anywhere else and they can play a part in your rehabilitation and body maintenance.

Note: Since magnets can cause skin irritation, it's best to give your skin a rest from them, perhaps while you sleep or when you're in the shower. If you do notice irritation, remove the magnets for a couple of hours to a day, and then reapply them.

Tennis Ball Massage

This is an oldie but a goodie. A tennis ball can be a source of great relief if you are experiencing tight, tense 'spasmed' muscles and here is how you use it:

- Put the tennis ball onto the carpet, or a rug

- Throw a towel over the ball in a single layer

- Now, lie on your back on top of the ball

- Move around on the ball to give yourself a massage in the painful and tense spots

- You can do it anytime, and you can do it yourself.

DON'T spend more than about 60 seconds in any one spot.

DON'T place the ball directly under the spine.

DON'T attempt to use this method below the buttocks or above the shoulders because it's just not effective.

DON'T increase pain.

Physical Manipulation Techniques

The objective of physical manipulation techniques is to move the various muscles, connective tissues, and vertebrae-into proper functional alignment. It is a very successful method and can often correct serious problems relating to stress and physical pain.

Any physical manipulation MUST always (without exception) be done by trained physical therapists. They are trained to recognize deficiencies or weaknesses in the biomechanics of any individual patient's anatomy and to work with people who have suffered injuries or surgery. Other than the physical manipulation they will usually also teach you certain stretches, exercises and techniques.

For example, a physical therapist will focus on stretching tight muscles and joints because without the ability to stretch, you naturally lose mobility. Furthermore, the stronger and more mobile you are, the more you have the ability to fight against any joint or muscle pain, and that applies just as much to the muscles and joints in your back as it does to any other part of your body.

Physical manipulation techniques that are used for the treatment of back pain include neuromuscular releasing, chiropractic, osteopathic, bodywork, and yoga.

Neuromuscular Releasing

Dr. Lewis uses a method known as neuromuscular releasing, a soft-tissue manipulation technique for releasing tissue texture alterations, such as knots, edema (excess fluid in body tissues), fibrosis (abnormal formation of fibrous tissue), and scarring, from various muscle tissue and from the layers between muscles.

The method involves using thumb pressure on the tissues in order to break up and release any tissue texture alterations that may be inhibiting muscle movement and contributing to pain.

Dr Lewis says: *"Following that, it is essential to relax and stretch these muscles out again, because it is generally my opinion that most dysfunction comes from excessive muscle tension rather than weak muscles.*

Muscles always work in pairs. When a muscle contracts, the antagonist to that muscle will be held in relaxation. For example, in order to lift something with your forearm, the biceps muscle will contract while the triceps on the opposite side of the arm must relax, otherwise we would simply tighten up and not be able to move at all.

59

In cases of low back pain, though, one of the most common things is to have a person do sit-ups to strengthen the abdominal muscles. Yet, quite often the abdominal muscles are not weak, but are being held in relaxation because the muscles in the back are in spasm. So if you can get these muscles in the back to relax, they will stop inhibiting the tone of the abdominal muscles."

Chiropractic Treatment

Chiropractic treatment is a very popular choice for reducing back and neck pain.

A visit to the chiropractor can be effective and apart from pain relief the manipulation also assists in realigning the body while the other treatment modalities are taking effect.

Chiropractic manipulation can in certain circumstances be every bit as effective as or even better than other medical treatment. But it is important to understand that chiropractic manipulation is not going to be effective in every situation.

Chiropractors specialize in the manipulation of joints and the vertebrae in the back and neck. Chiropractic theory holds that back pain is often due to misaligned vertebra that can press on a nerve and produce pain in the back and/or neck and other areas fed by the affected nerve.

Chiropractic treatment has been found to be more beneficial to patients with persistent back and neck complaints than other forms of manipulation. Research in Great Britain found chiropractic to provide *"worthwhile, long-term benefits"* for patients with low back pain in comparison to hospital outpatient management. This study also found chiropractic benefits to persist for a three-year period, indicating a long-term enhancement of health. For patients with uncomplicated, acute low back pain, chiropractic has also been found to be effective.

Finally, a cost comparison study of back-related injuries showed the number of work days lost for patients treated with chiropractic to be nearly ten times less than that of patients treated under conventional medical care.

Chiropractic treatment might have some good side effects as well; according to **Robert Blaich, D.C., of Los Angeles, California**, patients with chronic lower back pain who undergo chiropractic for some other problem like headaches or digestive problems often find that, in the course of treatment, the lower back pain goes away as well. Dr. Blaich states that since lower back pain frequently has to do with basic misalignments of the pelvis and spine, chiropractic is a particularly appropriate treatment. As he explains, *"Almost all forms of chiropractic involve correcting misalignments, which in turn reduce the stress on joints, help to reduce wear and tear on joints, and help to minimize joint deterioration."*

Dr. Blaich contends that chronic lower back pain usually stems from a preexisting weakness. At a minimum, he advises chiropractic treatment every three to six months, although many people benefit from more frequent visits to maintain proper alignment and safeguard against injury to intervertebral disks.

The frequency of visits depends on a myriad of predisposing factors, including the condition of one's body and lifestyle. As Dr. Blaich puts it, *"When you own a car, you wouldn't go 200,000 miles without getting your tires aligned. And if your tires were wearing out prematurely, you would replace the shock absorbers. With alignment, your tires will wear better. That is very similar to what we do in chiropractic as preventive maintenance for the back."*

Osteopathic Treatment

Leon Chaitow, N.D, of London, England says there is a wide range of osteopathic manipulative approaches for back pain, allowing patients the opportunity to choose among different options in order to find the one most appropriate for their specific needs.

Osteopathic techniques are being used to address chronic and acute back pain, as well as joint or soft-tissue problems.

The osteopathic techniques range from gentle joint mobilization to specific thrust methods similar to those used in chiropractic. The difference between osteopathic and chiropractic methods lies in variations in basic concepts, as well as in the forms of manipulation most commonly used.

While some osteopaths may manipulate the spine and other joints of the body to relieve back pain and restore alignments, they are also licensed to give injections in order to relieve painful inflammation in the joints. Additionally, they may apply electrical stimulation and various forms of mechanical therapy in order to trigger muscle relaxation, including gentle "muscle energy" techniques, and functional and positional release techniques, all unique to osteopathic medicine.

Bodywork

Bodywork is a combination of all the various forms of massage, deep tissue techniques, energetic light touch, Rolfing,

Hellerwork, Feldenkrais, the Alexander Technique, movement awareness therapies, energy healing, such as acupressure, shiatsu, and reflexology all of which can be applied to the treatment of back and neck pain.

Rolfing and Hellerwork are two of the more common forms of bodywork used for back pain and postural problems. Both these techniques involve the strenuous manipulation of the muscles, connective tissue, and joints to realign the body, muscles, and connective tissue.

Movement awareness therapies such as the Feldenkrais Method and the Alexander Technique have also proved effective for realigning and correcting posture.

These methods use light touch as well as visualization and suggestion to reprogram a proper posture and movement. These techniques are often able to greatly alleviate back and neck pain.

There are many other hands-on techniques that effectively treat back pain through energy healing, such as acupressure, shiatsu, and reflexology.

Invertors

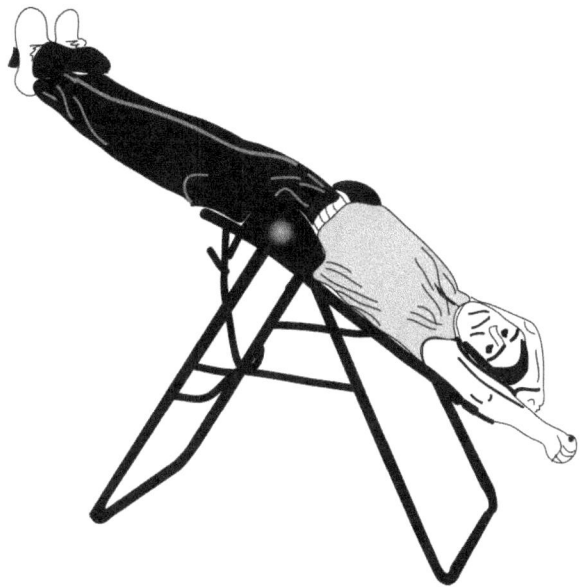

Invertors are devices that allow you to use your own body weight to help put traction on your spine.

The purpose of devices like invertors is to de-compress your spine and to stretch your muscles which are all good things to do but only if you doctor says so.

If used correctly an inversion machine can help you a lot. But it's not mandatory to have one to cure your back pain and it certainly is not good for all cases of back pain.

Warning: Please be careful. These devices, known as back swings or anti-gravity machines need to be approached with caution. You cannot just jump on one of these machines when you have back pain and hope it will be a cure all. Inversion is very bad in certain cases and you should never ever use an inversion machine without very specific instructions from your doctor.

Dr. Lewis also counsels his patients on a variety of home therapies for relieving back pain, including slant boards, inversion boots for hanging upside down, and back swings. *"All these devices apply some sort of traction to the tissues in the back,"* Dr. Lewis says, *"and that can be very helpful."*

Dr Lewis also says: *"Another important tool is shoe lifts for correcting any anatomical leg-length problems. I tend to be very aggressive about using shoe lifts, especially if the patient is young. … and I rarely find that they produce any negative response for the patient. They may be sore as their body adapts to the change, but in almost all cases I find it very, very positive."*

"Orthotics, which help to correct flat-footedness plus other inversions and eversions of the foot, are also helpful for back pain, as they correct and balance the foot, which is the foundation of all good posture" according to Dr. Lewis.

High-Tech Rejuvenation of the Back and Neck

Alternative Medicine: The Definitive Guide; Second Edition reports about the following high tech treatment option through the use of MedX machines:

MedX machines are unique, computerized back- and neck-strengthening devices that have been widely studied in a university setting. They were developed by Arthur Jones, the inventor of Nautilus exercise equipment. A three-minute MedX workout twice a week for several weeks can alleviate back pain and prevent back injuries, and a recent study indicates that the MedX might even help avoid back surgery. In the study, 60 patients who were surgical candidates did resistive extension exercise on the MedX; of the 46 participants who completed the program, only three required surgery.

The MedX works by strengthening the muscles of the back and increase the range of motion, both of which have been found to decrease back pain. While exercising the lower back, the MedX restraints inhibit the use of the pelvis and legs.

"This is key, since the major extensors of the back are the buttocks muscles and hamstring muscles," says Marc Darrow, M.D., Los Angeles, California. *"The muscles surrounding the*

vertebrae are usually weak even when the gluteus and hamstring muscles are strong. Once these muscles are strengthened and range of motion is increased with MedX, pain diminishes."

A case history involving tennis pro Jim Pugh illustrates the benefits that MedX can provide.

Pugh came to Jason Kelberman, D.C, one of Dr. Darrow's colleagues, suffering from low-back pain that had plagued him for three months, leaving him unable to play or teach tennis. Dr. Kelberman determined that his restricted range of motion and diminished strength were consistent with degenerative disc syndrome. After only three sessions of chiropractic adjustments Kelberman was able to significantly reduce Pugh's pain, at which point he had Pugh begin a strengthening program using the MedX. The result was that Pugh's strength quickly improved and he was able to again play tennis at competitive levels.

The Weightlessness of Aquatherapy Works like Magic

Aqua therapy is where exercises are carried out in water.

When you are submerged in water, you become near weightless, and it is far easier to exercise without putting strain on your body or applying pressure to your muscles.

Aquatherapy is excellent to work painful back muscles in order to loosen them and strengthen them in a non-impact environment.

Ultrasound and Other Energy Medicine

A high energy sound wave is used to help repair damaged muscles and bones while relieving the pain at the same time.

Dr Lewis says: *"Ultrasound helps to break up local edema as well as local fibrosis where there's been inflammation. Also, if there has been an injury and some kind of scarring between the muscle layers, the ultrasound can break that up to a certain extent. It will also warm the tissues, which helps to relax the muscles. It can reduce the nerve conduction velocities, which means that the rate at which a pain impulse travels along a nerve pathway to the brain is slowed down, causing a pain-relieving effect."*

Devices such as the TENS (Transcutaneous Electrical Nerve Stimulator) are also used for the relief of back pain. The TENS, which can be used at home, works by applying a small electrical current to the affected nerves in the area of the back pain, causing conduction to be blocked and pain to be relieved.

TENS units and other similar energy devices are also

believed to stimulate the production of endorphins, the body's own natural painkillers. Microcurrent electrical stimulators such as the Alpha-Stim and Micro-Stim may be more effective for long-term use than the standard amperage TENS units.

Back and/or neck pain can also be relieved by using infrared light or soft (cold) laser devices either on the back or on related acupuncture points.

Devices like the LightBeam Generator that photomagnetically break up the congestion in the lymph vessels of the back, abdomen, and pelvis can dramatically improve back pain, especially if used in conjunction with manual lymph drainage, dry skin brushing, or rebounding exercise.

Prolotherapy Produces Amazing Results

Alternative Medicine: The Definitive Guide; Second Edition reports as follows about prolotherapy:

Prolotherapy, also known as regenerative therapy or sclerotherapy, is a technique that can dramatically reduce or eliminate back pain. The technique involves the injection of a proliferant such as dextrose (small quantity of diluted sugar water) with local anesthetic into the area of pain in order to stimulate the body's natural healing processes via the production of collagen, which strengthens the weakened area and reduces pain.

One of the most prominent proponents of prolotherapy is former **U.S. Surgeon General C. Everett Koop, MD.** When he was 40 years old, two separate neurological clinics diagnosed him as having incurable back pain, which radiated down his leg. His pain, however, was completely relieved by prolotherapy, which was basically unknown to modern medicine at the time. Because of his own healing, he used prolotherapy for the remaining 20 years that he practiced medicine.

"Although patients may have had back pain for several years, one to four prolotherapy treatments is often enough to relieve their pain," Dr. Darrow says. *"If there is improvement after four treatments, the injections will be continued, usually to a maximum of eight times."* One of Dr. Darrow's patients, a noted football player Johnnie Morton, Jr., of the Detroit Lions, had back injuries and pain that persisted for ten years. *"After only two prolotherapy treatments, he had his first pain-free season,"* Dr. Darrow reports.

Another of Dr. Darrow's patients was a 61-year-old retired U.C.L.A. emergency room nurse, who came to him with a 15 year history of low back pain. Prior to her first visit, she had spent the previous month in bed taking pain medications prescribed by her doctor, who referred her to Dr. Darrow as a last-resort effort to control her pain.

When prolotherapy was explained to her, she said, *"The idea that a series of dextrose injections could take away my pain and possibly keep it from reoccurring sounded like a fairy tale to me. To my surprise, I was pain free after the first injections and have remained that way."*

Prolotherapy is not limited to treating back pain or injuries, but is applicable to all musculoskeletal pain problems including arthritis and headaches, Dr. Darrow points out.

Mind/Body Medicine

Psychoneuroimmunology (PNI) is the study of the interaction between emotions, the nervous system, and the immune system. In other words it is a study of the connection between mind and body.

Dr. Bresler acknowledges this connection between mind and body and uses a combination of guided imagery, relaxation, and biofeedback to help his patients.

In the case of treating back pain, his patients are encouraged to form an image about what's going on in their backs. He says: *"They give the pain a voice, asking it, 'What do you want? Why are you here? What do you have to offer? The pain may indeed have something to offer, like not going to work or not having to make love to one's spouse. When we get an answer, we ask it if there's a way the patient can get what he or she needs without having a painful back. In this way, we honor the body's inner wisdom and intelligence."*

Biofeedback is another such technique that works with the connection between the body and mind which teaches patients how to consciously control heartbeat, respiration, muscle tension, and brain waves. By using this technique, it is possible to learn how to consciously relax muscles and improve blood flow to the tissues in the back that are causing one to experience pain.

Melvyn Werbach, M.D., past Director of the Biofeedback Medical Clinic, in Tarzana, California, tells the following story of a mother of two infants who was suffering from chronic back pain. *"She had gone through two failed spinal fusions and lifting two babies put her in agony. We used Biofeedback-Assisted Relaxation Training (BART) and it was very successful, far more so than the surgery. Most of the pain disappeared and the rest she was able to* control. *Several years later, her back pain was still under control. BART seems to affect the immune system and other functions and it can lower the perception of pain."*

Dr. Darrow teaches his patients that back pain may be a way of handling other uncomfortable issues. *"Why is it that, a generation ago, many patients were hospitalized with gastric ulcers and instead, today, we find an epidemic of back pain?"* Back pain may be from subtle or overt emotional, mental, unconscious, or spiritual issues that can rapidly disappear once they are properly dealt with and resolved."

Acupuncture and Traditional Chinese Medicine

Traditional Chinese Medicine (TCM) says there is no such thing as simple back pain; there are several types of back pain. Every individual back pain is classified and differentiated. So while acupuncture is widely recognized as being an effective treatment for back pain, the specific acupuncture points that would be used by a specialist would depend upon the type of pain from which you are suffering.

Dr. Bresler says: *"Many studies have shown the effectiveness of acupuncture for treating back pain. At U.C.L.A., we researched the different styles of acupuncture, comparing*

Korean, Vietnamese, Japanese, Chinese, and American acupuncturists, and found them equally effective."

Dr. Maoshing Ni, D.O.M.,Ph.D., L.Ac., President of Yo San University, in Marina del Rey, California. says that *"acupuncture works to release the stress that has been internalized into the body."*

Back pain caused by pinched nerves can be treated with acupuncture, which helps to restore the flow of blood and energy that is needed to bring essential healing nutrients, such as calcium and magnesium, to the injured back.

"Acupuncture can also relax muscle spasms or strengthen weak back muscles," states Dr. Ni.

Dr. Eugene Kozhevnikov, M.D., O.M.D., of St. Petersburg, Russia, uses acupuncture to relax muscles and muscle contractions caused by damaged organs. Dr. Kozhevnikov claims that 90% of herniated disc cases should be treated with acupuncture first rather than undergoing surgery. His treatment involves electro-acupuncture, physical manipulation, and various energy medicine devices.

TCM holds the belief that when you have pain or discomfort, it is because your body balance and harmony is upset.

Consequently, in order to reduce or remove pain, it is necessary to restore balance and harmony and acupuncture is one of the primary methods used.

Most of us are not using (i.e. stretching and contracting) all of our muscles properly and that as a direct result of this, many of our muscles have contracted and tightened.

This contraction and tightening means that Qi (energy) and blood cannot flow through the muscles and when strain is placed on the muscle it will go into spasm.

An acupuncturist will treat your back and/or neck pain on the basis of moving blood and Qi around your body with the use of needles. A trained acupuncturist knows that there are many different blood and Qi 'channels' in your body, so their first task will be to examine various parts of your back to establish where the major centre points of pain are.

Your acupuncture practitioner will apply needles in both a local (i.e. at the point of pain) and distal (i.e. in other parts of the body) manner in order to open up your Qi channels. Don't worry, although needles are used in the process it is a very gentle process and not painful or uncomfortable at all. Most of the times you won't even feel the needles.

In modern times more and more practitioners are using an electric current rather than needles to stimulate the body and open the appropriate Qi channels and this is often a more attractive alternative for people who fear needles.

A study conducted by two leading Swedish doctors in 2002 about the effectiveness of acupuncture published in **'The Clinical Journal of Pain'** and reported on the Acupuncture Today website reports the following:

- According to the results, the two doctors tested acupuncture as a back pain treatment on a group of people who had been suffering from chronic lower back pain for at least six months.

- Every one of these people had tried various other back pain relief treatments or cures but to no avail.

- The test group was split into three smaller groups. The members of one of these subgroups received acupuncture treatment once a week for eight weeks, the members of the second group received electro-acupuncture, and the members of the third subgroup were given a placebo.

- The final results of the test indicated that all of the patients who had received acupuncture reported 'significant' improvement in their condition one month, three months and six months after completion of the treatment. They also reported that they were able to sleep more soundly than previously, and that they were also able to achieve higher activity levels than previously.

There seems to be little doubt that acupuncture as a treatment for back pain can be extremely effective although the test did report that there were certain types of back pain and patients that responded to treatment better than others.

Perhaps most interestingly, the study also indicated that both forms of acupuncture (using needles or electro-acupuncture) were equally effective.

Naturopathic Medicine

It is critically important to provide nutritional support for strengthening and repairing the tissues to relief inflammation. The nutritional support comes from following a healthy diet as well as consuming certain beneficial Vitamins, minerals and herbs.

Nutritional supplementation and support can play a major role in prevention and treatment of back and neck pain. Let's have a look at just a few everyday examples:

- When you sweat you tend to lose minerals and trace elements from your body, and if these minerals are not replaced you may suffer muscle pains and cramps.

- A lack of both sodium and potassium can cause cramps and pain, but both can be replaced relatively quickly. Sodium can be ingested in bouillon (beef or chicken would be best, but a vegetable bouillon would also work), while bananas are a tremendous source of potassium.

- Milk and milk-based dairy products are high in calcium, and calcium is essential for healthy bones and muscles. You should therefore drink a minimum of three glasses of milk a day if you are not taking on board sufficient calcium from other sources. This is particularly true of women who suffer back pain as a result of muscle strains or damage.

- Depending upon the cause of your back pain, even plain water can be beneficial. This is especially true if your pain is as a result of fluid depletion following exercise, but even if this is not the case, drinking water can help to alleviate back pain.

Let's have a closer look at the various foods, supplements and herbs that can help you to relief back and neck pain.

The Anti-Inflammation Diet to Relief Back and Neck Pain

Many of the leading health organizations like **the Arthritis Foundation** and the **American College of Rheumatology** have for decades been denying that diet can cure arthritis and/or inflammation. In fact they have been describing it as quackery.

On the other hand, alternative health practitioners have for almost 100 years been saying that diet could and in fact do fight inflammation. In recent times the conventional health practitioners are being overwhelmed with evidence to substantiate this fact.

Researchers have amassed data from 1911 showing that diet programs could and in fact do produce remission of inflammatory reactions in the body.

It has been found that certain foods contain allergens that irritate the body which it constantly have to fight and adapt to. Some of these allergens occur naturally in certain foods while others occur in the food additives. Some of the most commonly known foods that cause inflammation are <u>wheat, corn, milk, dairy products and red meat</u>. Common allergens like casein (in dairy products) and gluten (in grains) are quick to spark the inflammatory cascade.

Nightshade is a huge problem: In addition to the allergens noted before, it has also been proven that the nightshade family of foods also contains these allergens and it is better to avoid them as much as you can in your diet. Nightshade foods include; Potatoes, Tomatoes, Eggplant (Aubergine), Bell peppers (green, red, yellow, cherry), Hot peppers (long & red, red cluster), Chili peppers, (basically all peppers, except, white and black pepper), Paprika, Tabasco, Belladonna (used in homeopathy) Cayenne pepper (capsicum) Pimento, Henbane, Mandrake, Jimson weed and Tobacco. Yes tobacco is a nightshade!

Allergic reactions can occur to one or many of the above. For people who are outright allergic to nightshade foods common symptoms are nausea, diarrhea, dizziness, inflammation, stiffness in the joints, migraines and weakness/fatigue.

Furthermore, lowering the fat intake in your diet significantly lowers the inflammation in your body and it is recommended that the elimination of animal and vegetable fats may be helpful.

The Omega-3 oils found in flaxseed oil and in cold-water fish, such as tuna, salmon, herring, trout, mackerel, sardines, and cod liver are excellent inflammation fighters. So is GLA (gamma-linolenic acid), an omega-6 oil that is present in primrose oil, borage oil, and black currant seed oil.

It was also found that people who follow a more "primitive" diet (in other words avoiding refined foods and food additives) than those who don't, have a much lower incidence of inflammatory diseases such as rheumatoid arthritis, heart disease etc.

Therefore, it is highly recommended that you limit or eliminate sugar, saturated fat, meats, and refined carbohydrates from your diet and to eat copious amounts of vegetables, olive oil, fresh fruits, whole grains and unrefined carbohydrates.

Here are the foods to avoid and the foods to eat:

Foods to Avoid:

- All nightshade

- Sugar

- Artificial sweeteners

- Processed foods

- Junk food

- Red meat

- Pork

- White bread and pasta

- Frozen and canned foods

Foods to Eat:

- Wild Salmon and other fish

- Nuts and Seeds- walnuts, flax and pumpkin

- Olive Oil and Canola Oil

- Soy

- Fruits- especially strawberries & blueberries

- Vegetables - especially leafy greens

- Oats and other whole grains

- Water

Always remember that olive oil is rich in vitamin E, a courageous and extremely efficient soldier in the war against inflammation. Olive oil also contains polyphenolic compounds that have been shown to have both anti-inflammatory and antioxidative effects. So, consuming olive oil instead of those other pro-inflammatory fats and vegetable oils will significantly reduce the inflammatory processes.

By now you know that if you eat anti-inflammatory foods regularly you can and will reduce inflammation in the body. Below is a list of anti-inflammatory and other healthy foods to help you create a healthy diet and bring a balance to inflammation in your body. Please take note that this is not a comprehensive list. I included it into this book as a starting point just to demonstrate to you the many food choices we have that are much healthier than the ones we sometimes choose.

Oils

Choose: All cooking should be done with Extra Virgin Olive Oil and/or Grapeseed oil and/or Canola Oil. Use Avocado Oil or Olive Oil for salad dressings.

Avoid: Sunflower, Safflower, Peanut Oil, Butter, Lard, Gravy, Cream sauce, Non-dairy creamers, Hydrogenated Margarine and Shortening, Cocoa butter, Coconut, Palm and Palm-kernel oils and any other oils except those mentioned above.

Vegetables

Choose: Green leafy vegetables, green and brightly colored vegetables, Bok Choy, Broccoli, Broccoli Sprouts, Brussels Sprouts, Cabbage, Carrots, Cauliflower, Chard, Collards, Fennel Bulb, Garlic, Green Beans, Green Onions/Spring Onions, Kale. Leeks, Olives, Spinach, Sweet potatoes, Turnip Greens

Avoid: Nightshade vegetables like Potatoes, Tomatoes, Eggplant (Aubergine), Bell Peppers (green, red, yellow, cherry), Hot Peppers (long & red, red cluster), Chili Peppers, (basically all peppers, except, white and black pepper), Paprika, Tabasco, Belladonna (used in homeopathy), Pimento, Henbane, Mandrake, Jimson Weed and Tobacco. Also avoid Coconut, Creamy sauces, Fried or Breaded Vegetables

Fruits

Choose: Acerola (West Indian), Cherries, Apples, Avocados, Black Currants, Blueberries, Fresh Pineapple, Guavas, Kiwifruit, Kumquats, Mulberries, Papaya, Raspberries, Rhubarb, Strawberries. Most berries are packed with anti-inflammatory phytochemicals and anti-oxidants.

Avoid: Canned fruit packed in heavy syrup

Protein

Choose: Cold water oily fish, Cod, Halibut, Herring, Oysters, Rainbow Trout, Salmon, Sardines, Snapper Fish, Striped Bass, Tuna, Whitefish, Skinless white-meat Poultry, Nuts, Eggs, Legumes and Seeds. When you do eat red meat, choose lean cuts of Bison, Venison and other Game Meats, or the lowest-fat cuts of Beef, preferably grass-fed beef. Soybeans, Tofu, and Soy milk are three great sources of proteins that may help to reduce your inflammation.

Avoid: Milk and Dairy Products, Organ meats, such as liver, Fatty and Marbled Meats, Spareribs, Processed meats such as Cold cuts, Frankfurters, Hot Dogs, Bacon, Fried Breaded or Canned Meats.

Carbohydrates and Fiber

Choose: Most of your carbohydrates should come from whole grains, vegetables and fruits. Whole grain products have lots of fiber which is an excellent inflammation fighter. Choose Whole-wheat flour, Whole-grain Bread (must be 100 percent whole-wheat or 100 percent whole-grain), High-Fiber Cereal, Brown Rice, Whole-Grain Pasta and Oatmeal

Avoid: Muffins (except bran), Waffles, Corn bread, Doughnuts,

Biscuits, Quick breads, Granola bars, Cakes, Pies, Egg noodles, Buttered popcorn, High-fat Snack Crackers and Chips.

Nuts & Seeds

Choose: Almonds, Flaxseed/Linseed, Hazelnuts, Sunflower Seeds (But never sunflower oil for cooking!), Walnuts and Pumpkin Seeds.

Herbs & Spices

Basil, Cinnamon, Cloves, Cocoa (at least 70% cocoa chocolate), Liquorice, Mint, Oregano, Parsley, Rosemary, Thyme, Turmeric.

Drinks

Your body needs water in the form of foods and beverages every day. Other good fluid sources include 100% fruit juices (with no preservatives), herbal teas (especially green tea) and vegetable juices.

Nutritional Supplements for Back and Neck Pain

Bone consists of protein, collagen and minerals. Muscle fiber consists mainly of protein with large quantities of minerals in the fluid inside the muscle. So it is just logical that nutritional deficiencies or imbalances in the building blocks will compromise the health and function of both bone and muscles which can obviously lead to back and neck pain.

Once it has been established that deficiencies are contributing to your back and/or neck pain it is essential to take the right nutritional supplements.

Here are some excellent guidelines from Alternative Medicine: The Definitive Guide; Second Edition: Larry Trivieri, JR Editor, Introduced by Burton Goldberg:

For Acute and Chronic Back and Neck Pain

Willow bark, feverfew, rosemary, and the enzyme protease are useful to ease inflammation. For additional support, include a multivitamin, multi-mineral, amino acid complex, and eicosapentaenoic acid (EPA) from fish oil.

For Degenerated Cartilage (Osteoarthritis)

- Glucosamine sulfate and glucosamine HCL are the building blocks of cartilage and connective tissue, which maintain strong and flexible joints.

- Other useful supplements and herbs include N-acetyl-glucosamine, bovine and shark cartilage, EPA, and antioxidants such as Pycnogenol, Coenzyme Q10 Devil's claw,

Cat's claw, Yucca root, and Vitamins C and E.

- Vitamin C and bioflavonoids are extremely important for strengthening the connective tissues, especially in smokers who have depleted their vitamin C resources, says Dr. Lewis.

- He recommends taking 2,000-3,000 mg of each daily, in divided doses throughout the day.

For Acute and Chronic Muscle Spasms

- Calcium, magnesium, and potassium supplements, as well as lobelia herb.

- Homeopathic topical creams containing calendula, arnica, and ivy extracts can relieve spasms.

- Calcium-magnesium supplements should be taken for muscle relaxation, particularly in instances where there's muscle spasm and twitching, Dr. Lewis adds.

- He recommends 500 mg of a calcium-magnesium supplement daily, preferably in a citrate form, because it allows for much better absorption.

For Acute and Chronic Inflammation

Protease enzymes (if no ulcer or gastritis is present),

bromelain (enzyme compound from pineapple), mucopolysaccharides (such as bovine and shark cartilage), EPA, evening primrose oil, and the herbs yucca root, Boswellia serrata, and wild yam can help ease inflammation.

Herbs for Back and Neck Pain

Research suggests that depression and stress can make pain worse. In other words chronic pain sufferers who also suffer from depression or stress will experience more pain than those who are not suffering from depression or stress. The same research suggests that substances which can calm and soothe your nervous system will therefore also help to relieve your pain.

Herbs that can reduce your stress levels are likely to be highly effective aids in your fight against back pain and include herbs such as skullcap, valerian, St John's wort, poppy, willow bark, angelica, cayenne, wild yam, motherwort, rose and lavender.

If you have chronic back pain, try to drink a few cups of skullcap infusion every day, or alternatively take a dozen or so drops of skullcap tincture every day.

Essential Oils

It has also been shown that essential oils extracted from peppermint, pine, rosemary, frankincense, ginger, cloves or juniper can be used as pain killers because every one of them has recognized analgesic (pain killing) qualities.

You can infuse one liquid ounce (30 milliliter) of base oil such as olive or coconut oil with 10-12 drops of any of these essential oils, shake well and then rub the oil on the skin in the area of pain. This will alleviate the pain and also reduce any swelling or inflammation.

Grape Seed Extract

Grape seed extract is derived from the seeds and skins of red grapes. It is a primary source of Resveratrol (a substance naturally created by certain vines, pine trees, peanuts, grapes, and other plants). There are lots and lots of research showing the many health benefits of Resveratrol. Amongst many other benefits is has been shown to stop pain, stop the growth of the bacteria that causes stomach ulcers that can lead to cancer, protect DNA, protect against skin cancer, and is used to treat many other conditions. Resveratrol also became the first-ever supplement known to activate a longevity gene; plus, it is thought to be the answer to the "French Paradox" (the reason why French people can eat so much fat and not get heart disease).

Bromelain

Bromelain is a group of enzymes found in pineapple juice and in the stem of pineapple plants. It is an outstanding anti-inflammatory agent and for this reason is very helpful in healing sprains and strains as well as muscle injuries and arthritis. When inflammation is reduced, blood can move more easily to a traumatized area, easing pain and speeding healing.

Boswellia

Boswellia, aka boswellin or "Indian frankincense," comes from a tree that grows in the dry hills of India. Research has discovered specific active anti-inflammatory ingredients in this herb called boswellic acids. These acids have been shown to significantly reduce inflammation by deterring inflammatory white cells from infiltrating damaged tissue and improving blood flow to the joints. It also blocks chemical reactions that set the stage for inflammation to occur in chronic intestinal disorders such as Crohn's disease and ulcerative colitis.

Aloe Vera

Aloe Vera is succulent plant belonging to the lily family that grows wild in large portions of the African continent. It has many therapeutic uses and is now commercially cultivated in the United States, Japan, and countries in the Caribbean and Mediterranean. Aloe reduce inflammation, decrease swelling and redness, accelerates wound healing, facilitates digestion, aid in blood and lymphatic circulation, as well as kidney, liver and gall bladder functions. It also contains at least three anti-inflammatory fatty acids that are helpful for the stomach, small intestine and colon.

Devil's Claw

The plant grows in the deserts of southern Africa and is named after the distinctively shaped tips of its fruits. Evidence suggests that devil's claw may provide relief from low back and neck pain:

- In a small study including 63 people with mild to moderate back, neck, and/or shoulder pain after four weeks of treatment with a standardized extract of devil's claw root provided moderate relief from muscle pain.

- In a larger study including 197 men and women with chronic low back pain, those who received daily doses of a commercialized devil's claw extract every day for a month reported experiencing less pain and needing fewer painkilling medications than those who received a placebo.

- Devil's claw may also reduce the need for analgesic and non-steroidal anti-inflammatory therapy in those with knee or hip osteoarthritis.

Ashwagandha

Ashwagandha (pronounced Ash-wah-gone-dah) is a small evergreen shrub, is widely cultivated in India and the Middle East for its medicinal properties and has been used by the Indian Medical System for more than 2,000 years.

Studies have shown that Ashwagandha has anti-inflammatory, anti-stress, and immune-boosting properties. Various chemical constituents of the herb have shown a number of therapeutic effects.

Because ashwagandha has traditionally been used to treat various diseases associated with nerve tissue damage related to the destructive molecules known as free radicals, some researchers speculate that the herb may have antioxidant properties.

Horse Chestnut Extract

The extract comes from the fruits of the horse chestnut tree (Aesculus hippocastanum).

In the 1800s, European doctors discovered horse chestnut extract could help treat varicose veins, hemorrhoids, and other disorders caused by fragile veins and sluggish circulation. Scientists discovered three (3) very beneficial active ingredients in horse chestnut:

- **Aescin** is the first active ingredient that reduces inflammation and tones up vein walls, allowing blood to flow back to the heart more easily. It accomplishes this by plugging up minute holes and microscopic leaks in the tiniest blood vessels, the venules, and in the capillaries. In reinforcing the strength of veins, horse chestnut is believed to also promote their elasticity and prevent swelling and long-term damage to them.

- **Saponins** the second active ingredient that have the ability to eliminate cholesterol and it acts as a type of natural cortisone which cures all kinds of inflammation, such as arthritis, rheumatism, bursitis, colitis, and other inflammatory conditions.

- **Flavones (Flavonoids) known as bioflavonoids**, is the third active ingredient. Apart from their excellent antioxidant activity, flavonoids are known for their ability to strengthen capillary walls, thus assisting circulation.

Yucca

The yucca plant grows in abundance throughout the Southwestern United States and Mexico and is used to treat inflammations caused by degenerative diseases like arthritis and rheumatism.

The yucca root and leaves have Saponins, similar to Horse Chestnut, which are used for inflammation and pain relief for arthritis and joint pain. It is also good for blood purifying and cleaning of the kidneys and liver.

Scientists found that yucca helped patients with osteoarthritis & rheumatoid arthritis block the release of toxins from the intestines, which tends to inhibit normal formation of cartilage.

Yucca is also rich in Vitamin A, B-complex, and Vitamin C and a good source of copper, calcium, manganese, potassium, and fiber. It's almost like taking a multi-vitamin.

St. John's Wort

St. John's wort (Hypericum perforatum), contains numerous therapeutic substances well-known in the treatment of mild to moderate depression. St John's Wort is also used to control PMS, Fibromyalgia and Chronic Fatigue (chronic disorders characterized by widespread musculoskeletal pain, fatigue, and multiple tender points that occurs in precise, localized areas, particularly in the neck, spine, shoulders, and hips), anxiety, stress, chronic pain, infections, hemorrhoids, and many other ailments.

St John's wort oil can be liberally rubbed into any area of your back in which you feel pain, and as it is a particularly effective treatment for muscular pain, this can be an extremely valuable antidote to chronic or acute muscular back and/or neck pain.

DL-Phenylalanine (DLPA)

DL-Phenylalanine contains the two essential amino acids L-phenylalanine and D-phenylalanine. Our normal diets do not supply enough Essential Amino Acids and we need to get more of it in through supplementation:

- Studies have shown that L-phenylalanine can elevate the

mood, making DLPA a useful agent in combating depression.

- DLPA can also be used to treat chronic pain since it boosts the body's natural pain-killing response.

- DLPA has been known to increase the body's natural pain-killing response.

Ginger Root

Ginger root has proven to be a natural spice that is also widely prized for its medicinal properties. Specifically, ginger may help to:

- Relieve nausea, combat motion sickness, reduce dizziness, limit flatulence, control chronic pain, ease the pain of muscle aches and rheumatoid arthritis, and minimize symptoms of the common cold, allergies, and other respiratory conditions.

- Boost the pumping action of the heart, prevent the formation of clots, reduce cholesterol levels, and fight inflammation.

Ginger not only helps reduce pain caused by inflammation it also helps you promote an all-around healthier lifestyle.

White Willow Bark

The bark of white willow (Salix alba) has been used in China for centuries because of its ability to relieve pain and lower fever. Early settlers to America found Native Americans gathering bark from indigenous willow trees for similar purposes.

- The salicylic acid in White Willow Bark lowers the body's levels of prostaglandins, hormone-like compounds that can cause aches, pain, and inflammation.

- While White Willow Bark takes longer to begin acting than aspirin, its effect may last longer and, it does not cause stomach bleeding or other known adverse effects.

- It is typically used to relieve acute and chronic pain, including headache, back and neck pain, muscle aches and menstrual cramps and also control arthritis discomforts.

In summary then, White Willow Bark is actually a safer and longer lasting form of aspirin.

Peppermint

Peppermint (Mentha piperata) is a naturally occurring hybrid of spearmint (M. spicata) and water mint (M. aquatica) and has been proven to have medicinal benefits.

- Peppermint oil acts as a muscle relaxant, particularly in the digestive tract, and it can also reduce the inflammation of nasal passages and relieve muscle pains.

- Peppermint is used to treat irritable bowel syndrome, ease nausea and vomiting, control flatulence and diverticular disorders, improve digestion and reduce heartburn, dissolve gallstones, reduce the severity of herpes outbreaks, fight bad breath, control muscle aches and chronic pain, clear congestion and cough related to colds and allergies, control mild asthma, and fight stress.

- It keeps chronic pain and muscle aches under control

Cayenne (Capsicum)

It is estimated that Native Americans have used cayenne (or red pepper) as food and medicine for at least 9,000 years. The hot and spicy taste is due to an ingredient known as capsaicin which has very powerful pain-relieving properties.

- Laboratory studies have found that capsaicin relieves pain by destroying a chemical known as substance P that normally carries pain messages to the brain.

- It has been shown in human studies to improve the migration of white blood cells to attack foreign microorganisms and toxins in the bloodstream.

- It alleviates inflammation and can break up the deposits that contribute to sciatica pain.

Yoga, Tal Chi and Qigong

Yoga breathing exercises and postures as well as the movements practiced in Tai Chi and Qigong have the potential to reduce much of the tension and stress that can contribute to back pain. These techniques are therapeutic and help with relaxation through gentle exercise, stretching, and meditation.

Dr. Mary Pullig Schatz, M.D., author of Back Care Basics says: *"When your attention is directed inward, your body receives messages that you are safe and secure and that it is appropriate to relax. So muscles relax, blood pressure drops, nerves are calmed, anxiety is decreased, immunity is heightened, and healing is enhanced."*

A regular yoga, Tai Chi, or Qigong regime can help to prevent back pain in the first place.

Yoga places great emphasis on body alignment which helps to alleviate pain because it is often the fact that people's bodies are forced into positions where it is not correctly aligned that causes back pain in the first place.

There are many reasons why yoga is likely to be far more effective as a form of exercise for alleviating or reducing your pain when compared to other forms of exercise:

- Deep, slow breathing naturally relaxes your muscles, which will obviously reduce the chances of suffering a muscle strain or sprain in the first place, and alleviate the pain if you have already caused a strain.

- On top of this, the poses are all about stretching all the muscles in your body, and this also makes it far less likely that you will suffer strains or muscle damage in the future.

- It can reduce the pain that you may already be suffering by making you more flexible and supple,

- It can also prevent back problems developing if you are not already a back pain sufferer.

Later on in the book we will be showing you some specific yoga and qigong routines that could be of great benefit to you to prevent and/or relief back and neck pain.

Posture, Symmetry and Balance

Without getting involved in an argument about the meaning of the words posture, symmetry and balance, for the purposes of this book and what I am trying to explain let's agree as follows:

- By "posture" I mean the form or position or shape of my body when I move or when I am not moving when I sit, walk, lift and sleep.

- By "symmetry" I mean the balance of the various components (muscles and/or limbs) on the left and right side of my body. Symmetry is defined in the Oxford Dictionary as; *'right proportion between the parts of the body, balance and harmony...repetition of exactly similar parts facing each other or a centre'.*

Posture

So in order to try and clarify that a bit more; when I keep my head slanted to the left side for an extended period of time my posture have been bad and as a result the symmetry (balance) between the muscles on the left side of my neck has become disturbed or out of sync with the muscles on the right side of my neck. I will in all likelihood end up with a pain in my neck

You will soon see that posture and symmetry are major and significant issues when it comes to back and neck pain.

You might remember that in the chapter "The Causes of Back and Neck Pain under the heading "Posture Plays a Major Role" I gave a detailed explanation of the importance of good posture and how bad posture can cause serious health issues including back and neck pain.

There is a right and a wrong way to <u>sit, stand, walk, lift, carry, sleep, work and play</u>. And it is important to understand that we do all these activities with the same degree of force on the left side as we do on the right or on the front as we do on the back.

Try and recall last time you saw a lot of people standing, for instance in a room. How many of them were not standing symmetrically? You will find that many people stand with their weight on one leg or leaning a bit backwards or forwards.

Symmetry

Symmetry (balance) is one of the most crucial elements in recovery and one of the most commonly overlooked issues in the diagnosis of pain's root causes and it is sad that so few people (including doctors) don't even know it or recognize it.

Once you understand and correct symmetry it will go a long way to relief your pain and in many cases (up to 80%) that might be the only treatment you need.

The important conclusion is that if **you lose symmetry you WILL end up in pain**. It's not a question of 'if' it's a matter of 'when'. On the other hand if you rectify symmetry you may get rid of pain.

A loss of symmetry usually gradually accumulates from bad posture, which brings us to the next important thing to remember; **loss of symmetry is caused by bad posture.**

Just look around you and observe when people move, walk, sit sleep and you will quickly see how many people have really bad postures, necks not straight and square on the shoulders, slouching when sitting on a chair, arching the neck and back forward when typing or writing etc.

Symmetry loss, if not addressed can have the effect of undergoing treatment, getting some temporary relief, but in a few days the pain is back as bad as ever.

The reason is, unless the underlying symmetry loss is dealt with, temporary relief is the best you can hope for.

When you know how and why, you can restore symmetry if the damage done is not beyond the point of no return. Even then, some progress is very often possible.

Remember no amount of treatment can rid you of pain unless it also addresses this loss of symmetry.

Here is a golden rule: **The right stretches WILL restore balance (symmetry).**

Our actions and posture throughout the day often result in a loss of symmetry, and stretching can restore it.

A Few Case Studies

Richard Convery, author of the books 'Back for Life' and 'My Necks Book') who has been helping countless people with back and neck pain for many years, describes how he encountered and fixed a few cases of lost symmetry:

Case study 1 – *"Another classic I remember was a man in his 70s. He had come to me after I had helped his wife and a bunch of her friends. He had the tightest right hamstring muscles (back of thigh) I had seen for many sleeps and had been suffering back pain for over 30 years.*

The interesting thing about this man was that he was, as I quickly discovered, an extremely determined character. I gave him a challenge and he met it head on, achieving symmetry and vastly reduced pain with quite outstanding improvement in mobility in less than six weeks.

Remember, he had been suffering severe pain and had been having treatment for over 30 years, yet he did the 'fixing' all by himself."

Case study 2 – "A lady in her 30s came to see me a few years ago with a problem that I was confronted with in about six out of every ten people.

You may well have heard of this condition - it's referred to as a short leg, or more correctly - a 'functional short leg'. I always ask people if they have ever fractured either leg as a fracture (particularly a complex fracture), can result in an 'actual' short leg, which is where there is an actual discrepancy in the bone lengths in the two legs. Her response was that she hadn't, so the next challenge was to find out WHY she had this 'functional short leg'.

The lady hadn't come to me with a problem with her legs, she came to me with - you guessed it already didn't you - a sore back!

Now this particular problem wasn't a problem of any noteworthy duration OR particularly difficult to rectify, though it was causing her a great deal of grief. The interesting thing here is... and what I want you to get a grip of... what happened when I gave her some stretches to do to correct her particular 'cause' of symmetry loss. She duly did as I asked and came back to see me STILL with a sore back. So I asked her what she had been doing.

"Well", she said, "I stretched the leg as you told me AND my back as well... but it didn't get any better".

Hang on, let's back up a bit..."What do you mean the leg?"

"Well, I knew I only had to stretch the 'short' one to make it the same length as the other one" WRONG!!!!!

When I examined her I discovered she had gone (in the space of four days), from having a 'functionally short' right leg to a 'functionally short' left leg. This (hopefully!) will send a loud and clear message to you that the imbalances in your body CAN change and can change QUICKLY. The challenge is to bring about the change we want and to produce the results we need. Once we sorted out that little hiccup, she was fine. SYMMETRY IS IMPORTANT!"

This case just demonstrates how critically important it is to always maintain the balance – in other words **whatever you do on**

one side of the body you have to do on the other.

Case study 3 – *"Another guy springs to mind. He was self-employed in the building industry, aged in his late 30s and had been having treatment for a bad back for over 20 years. An interesting challenge for very different reasons, he had what could only be described as a unique view of life. He was significantly asymmetrical (ie, NOT symmetrical), and had a 'functional short' left leg.*

This was predominantly due to years of working in crouched positions, climbing on work sites and using heavy power tools.

He regained SYMMETRY over a period of two months. The duration of his recovery was largely due to two main reasons; firstly, the demands of his very physical work and secondly, an attitude that – initially - questioned the validity of what I was telling him. After all, HE'D BEEN TREATED BY EXPERTS!

What is so satisfying about this particular man is that I met him years later and he declared with unbridled pride that he had been pain-free ever since and was spreading the word to 'stacks' of his friends."

Posture Comes First

From the previous chapter it should be clear that posture causes loss of symmetry and therefore it is just logical to start by correcting any posture issues. So how do you know if you have a posture issue? The easiest way is to ask someone to observe you and tell you and obviously it is good to also "listen" to your body.

Dr. Pamela Adams, D.C., a chiropractor and yoga instructor in Larkspur, California says: *"Your body is always giving you messages. 'This position hurts,' 'Get up and stretch,' 'Time to quit and rest.' If you ignore the messages-if you 'go through the day living between the top of your head and your chin,' you won't be aware of your back pain until it's acute, with much more severe symptoms, and it will be much harder to fix."*

Here's her advice:

- Set an alarm to go off every hour while you're awake. For 15 to 30 seconds after the alarm sounds, consciously notice how your body feels. (If you're already in pain, make this "appointment with your body" every 15 minutes.)

- Are you sitting correctly? If not, lift your breastbone.

- Are your shoulders up around your ears? Lower them.

- Pretty soon, checking on your body throughout the day will become automatic, and you won't need the alarm.

How to Sit

Dr. Pamela Adams says: *"One of the main culprits in chronic, non-traumatic lower-back pain is sitting and leaning back. Leaning back flattens the lower, or lumbar, area of your back, depriving the lower back of its natural curve. The weight of your body then pulls down on the lower lumbar vertebrae in the spine, stressing the ligaments and disks. After many years of sitting this way, you may develop lower back pain."*

Leaning back while sitting also puts your weight in the middle of your buttocks, right where your sciatic nerve passes into your legs. *"If you sit this way year after year, you may pinch your sciatic nerve, and you'll start developing shooting pains down one or both legs,"* Dr. Adams warns.

Practicing correct posture, she says, is an effective way to prevent and relieve muscular back pain. And it's easy to do in any situation.

How to Sit On a Chair

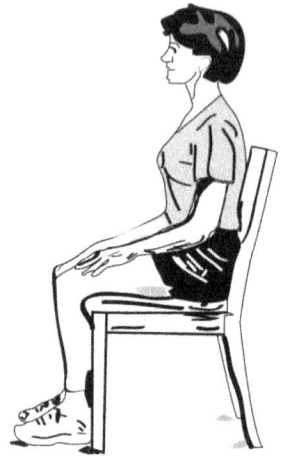

Dr. Adams says:

- *"The proper position for sitting is "just a smidgen" in front of your "sit bones," or the ischium bones of the pelvis. Those are the big bones that you can feel pressing against the chair right where your thighs end and your buttocks begin. At least, you can feel them when you are sitting correctly.*

- *Lean slightly forward from your hips, then, keeping your pelvis in place, move your upper back slightly back.*

- *That means don't slouch forward, don't round or hunch your back and shoulders, and keep your feet flat on the floor. You should be conscious of the curve in the small of your back," she says.*

- *The key to this pain-relieving, pain-preventing sitting posture is to lift your breastbone as you sit.*

  - *Pretend that a string is attached to the middle of your chest and is nudging your breastbone upward.*

  - *You want to lengthen the space between your belly button and your breastbone.*

  - *This 'corrected' sitting posture will feel awkward for a few days, however, because sitting incorrectly for so long can change the configuration and tone of your muscles.*

- *Do this breastbone-lifting exercise whenever you notice that you are leaning back or slumping over.*

- *The resulting posture not only will position your body correctly on your sit bones it will also position your head correctly on top of your spine, putting your spine in a natural alignment that supports your musculature and gives the overworked muscles of your lower back some much-needed relief.*

How to Sit When Driving

Dr Adams says: *"Many people who drive for a living have terrible back pain. That's because car seats seem designed to hurt your back. . Your knees are higher than your hips, throwing the weight of your body onto your sciatic nerve. And you're leaning back with your head forward and your arms extended, which stresses your lower back (and your neck)."*

Here is how she says you can minimize the damage:

- *"Your car seat should be as flat as possible so that your knees and hips are at the same level. You want to drive the same way you sit.*

- *If your car seat doesn't adjust automatically, you can build up the dip in the seat by sitting on a folded towel, a foam wedge, or a small pillow.*

- *Put a small pillow behind your lower back as well.*

- *Next, position the seat so that you aren't reaching for the steering wheel or leaning forward to grasp it. The wheel should be close enough that your arms can hang naturally from your shoulders and your shoulders feel relaxed.*

- *Just be sure that your breastbone is about 10 inches from the center of the steering wheel. That way, you'll lessen the*

possibility of injury from your seatbelt or airbag if you're in an

accident."

How to Stand

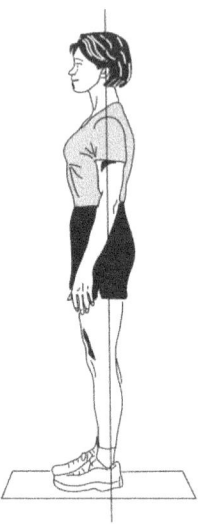

Dr. Adams says: *"For pain-free posture when you're standing, do the breastbone-lifting exercise, then have a friend look at you from the side. If you're standing correctly-that is, in a posture that can prevent or relieve back pain-a vertical line could pass directly through your ear, the middle of your shoulder, the middle of your hip bone, and the outside of your ankle bone."*

"Correcting posture-induced back pain is very logical and very simple," says Dr. Adams, *"but people make it so difficult. The body is a perfect mechanism. All we have to do is remove whatever imbalances are in the way of the body performing the way it is supposed to-and this easy exercise does just that."*

How to Always Lift Any Object

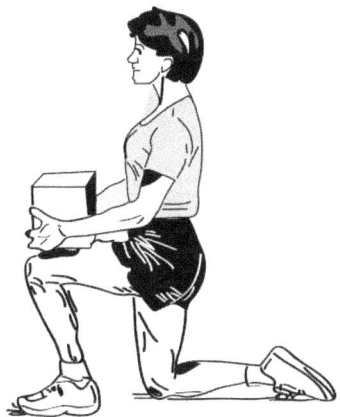

- Never ever bend over at the waist.

- Squat with your knees apart, with the object between your knees and as close as possible to your body. Using your legs, stand up and lift, bringing the object closer to your body as you stand. Be sure to keep your back straight.

- If you can't manage a squat put one knee on the floor, then, using your arms, move the object onto your opposite thigh and, with a firm grip on the object, simply stand up.

How to Sleep

Sleep time can be a chance to realign a back that's been stressed all day, says Dr. Adams. Here are two tips from her:

On Your Back

- Don't sleep on your side. Sleeping on your side puts your head forward, hunches your shoulders, and collapses your chest area, which means that your back can't extend and arch. When you sleep on your back the body opens up and you stretch, extend, and lengthen your back.

- Also, sleep with a thin pillow so that your head is not pushed too far forward.

- Shape the pillow so that it fits comfortably under your neck, making it thinner under your head and thicker under your neck for support. You should also put a folded or rolled towel in the small of your back for support, says Dr. Adams. The thickness of the towel depends on your body. It should be a little uncomfortable, but not much.

- If you're pregnant, however, don't sleep on your back after the first trimester. As an alternative, she suggests lying on your side, but not in the fetal position. Align your spine as best you can, then use a pillow that's as high as the distance between your shoulder and your neck so that it can support your head without pushing it too high or letting it sag.

On Your Stomach for Sciatica

Dr. Adams says: *"For years, people have been told that they should never sleep on their stomachs if they have bad lower backs. If you have sciatica, though, that could be bad advice.*

Sciatica is caused by overstretching ligaments and muscles in the back until they're pressing on the sciatic nerve. It's usually marked by shooting pains down one or both legs and is a condition that should be checked by a doctor.

If you sleep on your stomach when you have sciatica, gravity can restore a natural curve to your back, relaxing those ligaments and muscles so the nerve can heal itself."

How to Look Down

Hope Gillerman, a certified instructor of the Alexander Technique (a type of movement and posture re-education) in New York City says:

"When most people look down, they bend from the middle of their upper backs, making their shoulders round. This puts a lot of body weight in front of your spine, making your neck and shoulders "grip" to keep you from falling forward.

Instead, keep your neck upright and look down by letting your nose and chin drop and the back of your neck muscles relax. Use the previous affirmations to soften your neck and widen your shoulders. This is really crucial for eliminating neck and shoulder pain. When people realize that that's all they have to do to look down, they say, 'Oh, that's so much easier on my neck and shoulders."

How to Talk on the Phone

Talking on the phone is an activity where people develop a lot of neck tension. The reason: You tilt your head to the receiver instead of keeping your head balanced and upright and bringing the receiver to your ear. You should bring the phone to your ear. If you have to talk on the phone a lot get a headset.

How to Brush Your Hair

When you brush your hair keep your head balanced and move your arms and the brush up to your head. Don't bend your neck.

How to Hold Your Shoulders

Shrug off the slouching. **Hope Gillerman** says: "*Maybe you've been told that your shoulder pain is caused by slouching. Well, that can worsen the pain but don't correct your posture by pulling your shoulders back. That tightens the trapezius muscles in your back, causing even more muscle pain and straining your neck, shoulders, and upper back.*

First, shrug your shoulders up and let them fall forward, then shrug them up and let them fall back.

Finally, shrug them up and let them fall in between. That's where you want to leave them just sitting there on top of your body. Think of them as large shoulder pads."

Stretching and Exercising is Not the Same Thing

Staying in the same position for extended periods of time, such as sitting at a desk, driving a car or standing while you are working, causes tense muscles, increased pressure on the nerves and shortened muscles. In order to avoid this you need to do some stretching.

Dr. Doug Lewis, N.D., past Chair of the Physical Medicine Department of Bastyr University, in Kenmore, Washington says: *"Without a doubt, stretching is far more important for the relief of back pain than strengthening exercises. We really focus too much on strengthening muscles and I think it's a mistake, until we've done a good job of stretching them."*

It is necessary that you understand the difference between stretching and exercising, as well as when and how to use them. Stretching and exercising are very different:

Stretching is ...

- The main purpose of stretching is to bring flexibility and train the muscle fibres to lengthen effectively and to restore symmetry in the body.

- Stretching is the **first thing** you should do when you wake up in the morning, the **last thing** you do at night and it should also be the very first thing you do **before** and **after** any exercise. Stretching is quick and it is easy.

- Stretching should be done every day and if possible several times a day.

Exercising is ...

- The main purpose of exercise is to train muscle fibers to shorten, to increase strength, to help achieve support and shape to the body.

- You always have to stretch before and after you have done exercises.

- Exercises should be done only once in every 48 hours (every two days)

Stretches and Exercise can be for Prevention or Therapy

I have categorised the stretches and exercises into "prevention" and "therapeutic".

Prevention type stretches and exercises will do just that - prevent the onset or reoccurrence of back or neck pain.

Therapeutic type stretches and exercises aim to cure/treat/relief back or neck pain.

**It has been proven that proper stretching and exercise routines, when done consistently, is the most permanent cure for chronic back and neck pain.**

Stretches for Pain Prevention and Posture

Below are four (4) sets of easy stretches you can do at work. These stretches will help prevent pain and discomfort and most importantly help you to establish and maintain good posture which will ensure no loss of balance/symmetry.

You can rotate the set you want to do every time or make up your own set, out of the various stretches described below and use it all the time. Just make sure that when you make up your own set of stretches below that you stretch all the important muscles in the neck, shoulders, upper and lower back.

For all stretches:

- No jerking and sudden movements ever.

- Move slowly and smoothly.

- Breathe normally.

- Stretch at least every two hours (preferably every hour) to relief muscle tension and improve posture and enhance your health and wellbeing.

- If you experience any pain whatsoever when doing any of the stretches stop it and consult with a doctor to find out what is causing it.

- Perform each stretch as shown, relax then repeat on the opposite side.

- Make sure to perform each stretch as shown, relax then repeat on the opposite side as required.

- Always remember it is essential that any muscle you are going to stretch must absolutely be relaxed.

Note: Please discuss these stretches with your doctor or a health professional if you have any injury or medical condition.

Prevention Stretches Set 1 - On Your Chair (2-3 Minutes)

Here is some general stretches you can do from your chair. These are very easy and quick to do. Do it slowly no sudden jerking movements and hold it for 30 seconds when you reach the desired position. It will take you about 2-3 minutes maximum.

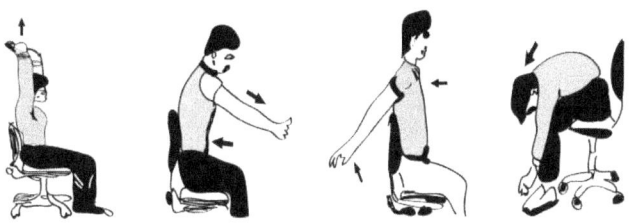

Prevention Stretches Set 2 – Next To Your Chair (4-5 Minutes)

This is a nice and easy set of stretches provided by Medibank Health Solutions which you can do at work. It takes only 4-5 minutes and you can do it 4 to 5 times a day. You will feel a lot better once you get into the habit of doing this.

The Lower Back

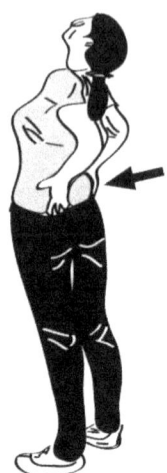

- Stand with feet apart

- Place hands on the back of your buttocks fingers pointing downwards

- Gently push the hips forward and downwards while exhaling and relaxing the buttocks

- Continue to push the hips forward while gently bending backwards to a point that feels comfortable for the back

- Hold the stretch for 5 seconds and repeat 10 times.

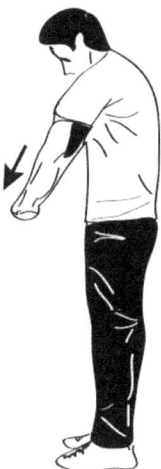

- Interlock your fingers in front of your body with palms facing outwards as shown

- Push your palms down towards the ground

- Gently pull your shoulder blades apart and bend head forward until a stretch is felt between the shoulder blades

- Repeat 5 times

Arm/Wrist Stretch

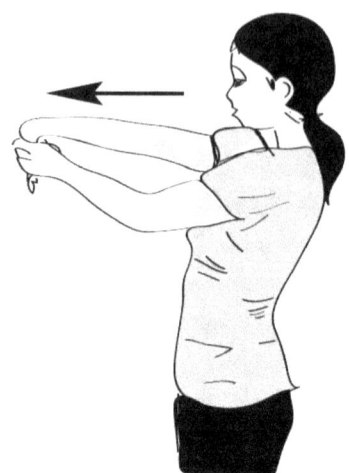

- Raise your right arm, with palm facing forward and fingers facing downwards

- Grasp the right palm with left hand as shown

- With wrist locked, gently straighten arm out in front of you until s stretch is felt in the right arm

- Now repeat for the left arm

- Complete 5 stretches with each arm

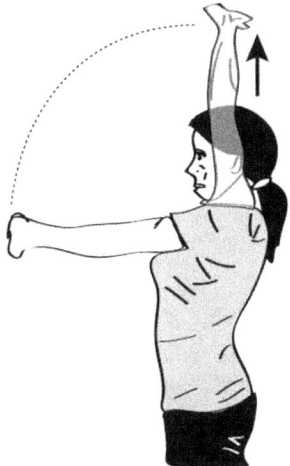

- Straighten your arms out in front of your body

- Interlock your fingers with palms facing downward as shown

- Raise arms to above your head reaching for the ceiling

- Do not arch your back

- Repeat 5 times

The Shoulders

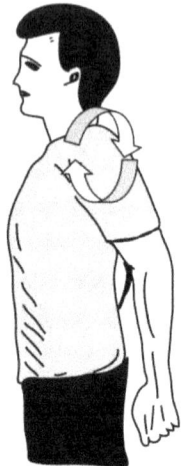

- Start with both your arms relaxed beside your body

- Slowly raise both shoulders toward your ears then roll the shoulders backwards in a circular movement, gently squeezing the shoulder blades together

- Repeat 4 times.

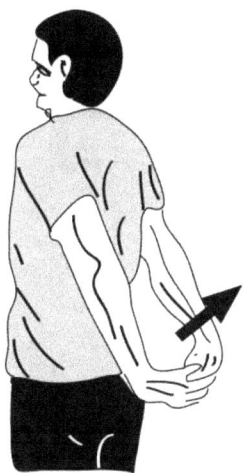

- Grasp your hands together behind your back, keeping your chest and head up as shown

- Gently squeeze your shoulder blades together while moving the arms back and up until a stretch is felt across the front of the chest and shoulders

- Repeat 4 times

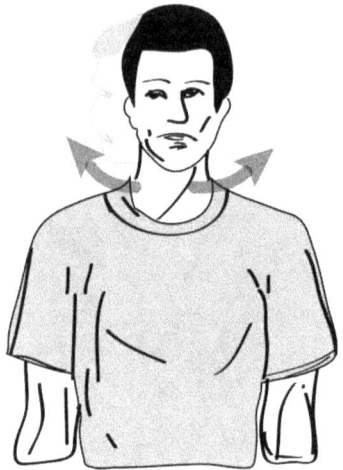

- Slowly turn your head to look over your right shoulder stretching the left side of the neck

- Then repeat to the left side stretching the right side of the neck

- Hold each stretch for 20-30 seconds

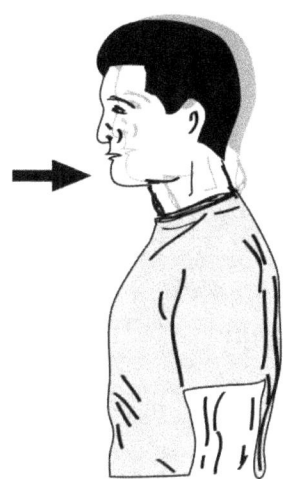

- Keep your head in the neutral position looking straight ahead

- Pull your chin backwards to align your ears with your shoulders

- Hold for 20-30 seconds

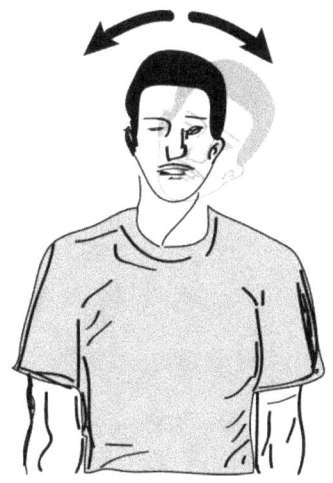

- Slowly drop your head towards your left shoulder stretching the muscles on the rights side of the neck

- Then repeat to the right side stretching the left side of the neck

- Hold for 20-30 seconds

Prevention Stretches Set 3 – On the Chair Again (2-3 Minutes)

Dr, Michael D. Pedigo, D.C, a chiropractor in San Leandro, California, and president of the American Chiropractic Association says:

"These three simple stretching exercises (all done while sitting in a chair) can keep your spine flexible and help prevent back pain. It's very important to do these exercises on an ongoing basis-even when you're pain-free-to counteract stresses and strains in the muscles of the back and prevent recurrent episodes of back pain."

Do them three times a day-in the morning, at midday, and in the early evening.

Don't worry if you hear some snapping and popping as your joints move through their full ranges of motion, as long as it causes no sharp pain. If it does, stop the exercise and see a chiropractor."

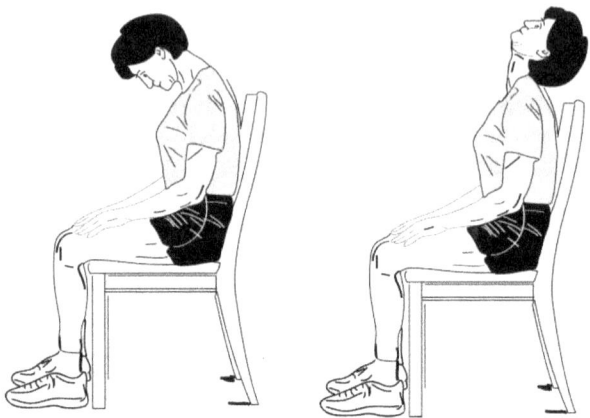

- Sit in a chair in a normal, upright sitting position with your legs hip-width apart and your hands on your knees.

- First, slowly lower your head toward your chest as far as you can without forcing it *(a)*.

- Then, in one smooth, continuous motion, slowly bend your neck back as far as you comfortably can *(b)*.

- Repeat this forward-and-back motion slowly 10 times in each direction, but do not force either motion.

Side- To-Side: Increasing Flexibility

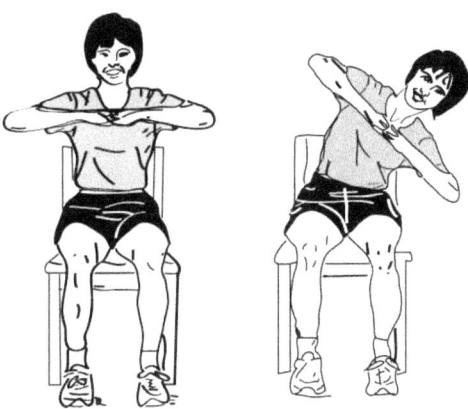

- In the same sitting position, hold your hands palms down in front of you and lace your fingers together.

- Point your elbows to the sides, horizontal to the floor (a).

- Slowly bend to the left from the waist, tilting so that your left elbow points toward the floor and bending your spine as far as you comfortably can (b).

- Return to the upright position and repeat on your right side.

- Do this 10 times in each direction. "Your spine should move like a willow tree"

Full Twist: For Your Whole Spine

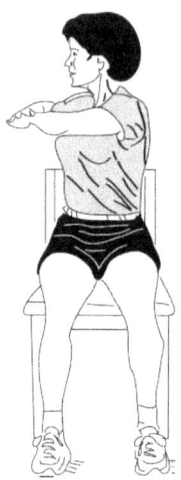

- In the same position, with your fingers laced and your elbows out, turn your head and shoulders to the right, letting your spine comfortably twist as far as it can.

- Repeat in the other direction.

- Slowly Do 10 twists to each side.

Prevention Stretches Set 4 - Relax the Neck Muscles (1 minute)

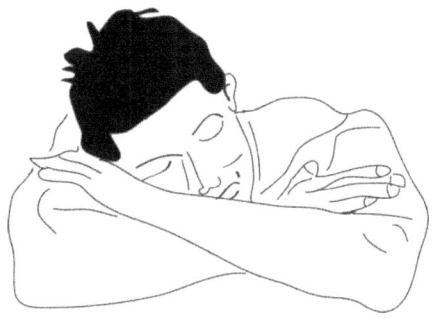

Fold your arms on top of each other genie-style and put them on the desk. Rest your forehead on top of your wrist; just let it sink into your arms, then feel your neck muscles relax do it on both sides for 30 seconds.

Therapeutic Stretches for Back Pain Relief

The various sets of stretches described and illustrated below are for therapeutic purposes. In other words these stretches are treatment for an existing condition and will help to cure or relief your pain.

You don't do all of these stretches you select one or more sets that is applicable to your condition and do that as described.

Therapeutic Stretches Set 1 – Lumbar Curve or Sway Back Routine

Dr. Doug Lewis, N.D says: *"If the muscles in both legs are tight, it can produce an anterior pelvic tilt, where the whole pelvis leans forward. This oftentimes creates a lordosis in the back, which is an excess amount of lumbar curve, commonly referred to as sway back."*

Dr. Lewis, N.D., describes a set of four easy stretches to treat and cure this condition:

Stretching the Rectus Femoris

One of the most common muscles associated with this kind of back pain is the rectus femoris, the muscle that runs from above the hip down through the kneecap and into the front of the tibia (the inner, longer bone of the leg between the knee and ankle).

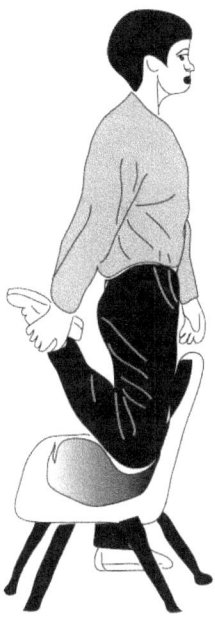

- Stand and put the knee of the leg you want to stretch on the seat of a chair, while holding the back of the chair with the opposite hand for balance.

- The idea is to pull the heel of the leg you want to stretch to the buttocks, and push forward with the pubic bone,"

- This will push the pelvis backward, and you'll feel the stretch all the way from the knee, up the leg, to the front of the thigh.

The Cat-Cow position

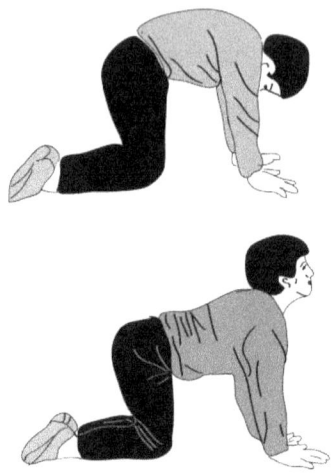

The "Cat-Cow" yoga position is where you're on your hands and knees, and you alternately drop your back into a sway back position, and then arch it like a cat. Do it slowly and in a controlled way.

The "Pelvic Rock"

This is done sitting in a chair.

- Sit up straight, back against the chair back so that you have the normal low back curve.

- Then allow your pelvis to roll back as if you were going to slouch into the chair.

- Hold that for a few seconds and then come back into the straight position with the normal lumbar curve.

Make Your Leg Longer

This is a very useful stretch especially when there is acute back pain, where you can't move much or when you are stiff in the morning and have trouble getting out of bed.

- While lying flat on your back, perhaps with a pillow under the knees so as not to strain the lower back, alternately push one foot out and then the other.

- You don't actually have to be pushing against anything.

- Rather, as you're pushing out with your heel, it's as if you're trying to make your leg longer.

- This rocks the pelvis back and forth instead of from front to

145

back as in the Pelvic Rock.

- As you do each stretch, hold the stretch, don't bounce. Hold it for 5-10 seconds, then release and relax for 5-10 seconds, then go back into the stretch for 5-10 seconds.

Therapeutic Stretches Set 2 – The RC Lower Back Pain Routine

This is an excellent set of stretches, from Richard Convery (Author of the books Back 4 Life and My Neck's Book), used by many people to cure back pain. It only takes 5 minutes in the morning before you get out of bed. I personally know of a large number of people who got tremendous benefit from this set of stretches.

- Do them every day for the rest of your life it will cure and prevent

- You MUST do them when you wake up in the morning before you get out of bed while to spine is decompressed and muscles are warm and relaxed

- It is very important to do the stretches in the order described below

- Do not change the order in which you do the stretches as you will injure yourself if you do

- Make sure that when you experience pain you stop immediately - never increase pain

- Do all stretches slowly and smoothly - no sudden or jerking movements

Rotate the Spine (60 seconds)

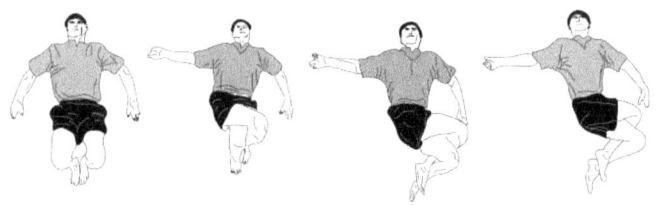

The purpose of this stretch is to rotate the spine. It is an excellent stretch and has been hailed by many as the Rolls Royce of stretches. The photos explain how you should execute it. Hold it for 30 seconds once you have reached your point of resistance. Then do the same one the other side holding it for 30 seconds as well.

Don't worry if you can't go down as far as it shows in the photos it will improve over time.

Lumbar Stretch (30 seconds)

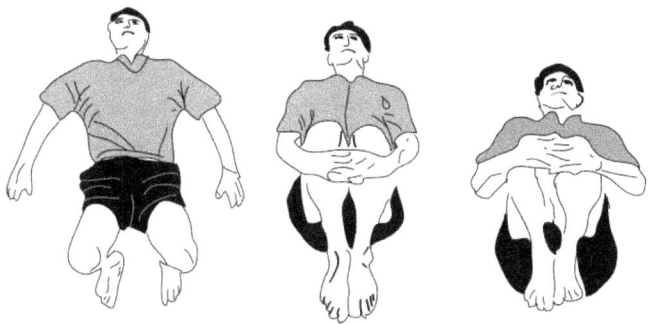

The purpose of this stretch is to improve and balance the forward and backward movement of the spine but with no weight on it. Hold it for 30 seconds once you have reached your point of resistance. Don't worry if you can't bend as much as it shows in the photos it will improve over time.

Side to side Spine Movement (30 seconds)

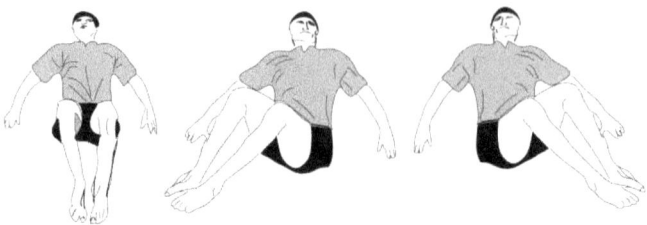

The purpose of this stretch is to improve and balance the side-to-side movement of the spine. This is a continuous movement from side to side with the lower back for 30 seconds. So you don't actual stretch the muscles as much as you move it side to side.

Pelvis Muscles (60 seconds)

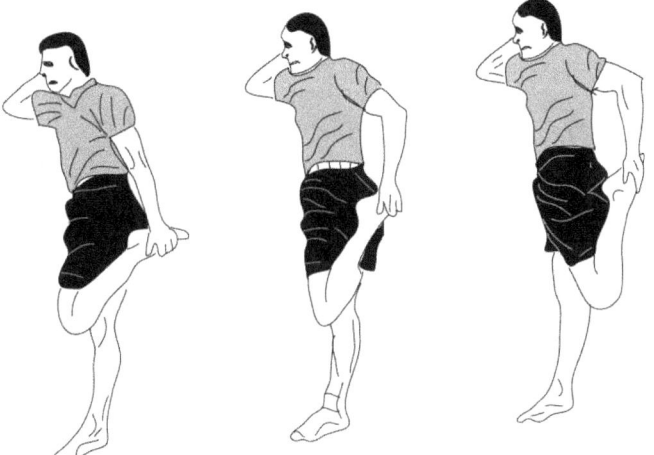

This stretch is extremely effective in the stretching of muscles that attach to the front of the pelvis. Lie on you side as shown in the photo, grab hold of your foot and slowly pull it up towards your bum as shown. Keep it there for 30 seconds then turn over and do the same on the other side.

Hamstring Stretch (60 seconds)

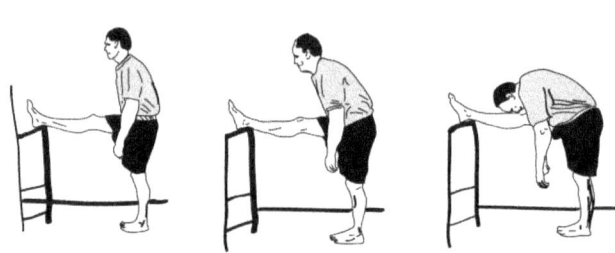

The purpose is to stretch the muscles in the lower back and the hamstrings. Hold it for 30 seconds once you have reached your point of resistance. Don't worry if you can't bend as much as it shows in the photos it will improve over time. Switch legs and do it for another 30 seconds on the other side.

Thigh and Hips (60 seconds)

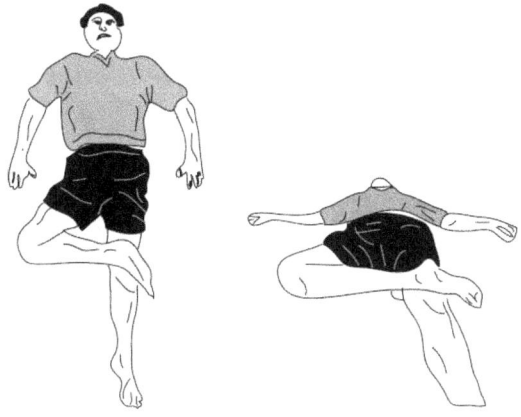

The purpose of this stretch is to stretch the muscles of the inner thigh and hips and to mobilize the knee joint. Hold it for 30 seconds once you have reached your point of resistance. Don't worry if you can't bend as much as it shows in the photos it will improve over time. Switch legs and do it for another 30 seconds on the other side.

Therapeutic Stretch Set 3 – Feldenkrais Relax and Balance the Entire Spine

Alternative Medicine: The Definitive Guide; Second Edition: Larry Trivieri, JR Editor, Introduced by Burton Goldberg provides the following stretch - a variation on a typical Feldenkrais exercise that can greatly benefit an aching back. It takes about 5 minutes to perform.

1. Lie on your back and take a few deep breaths. Notice how your spine is resting on the floor.

    a. Do all the vertebrae touch or are there spaces between your back and the floor?

    b. Does one side of your back touch the floor differently than the other?

    c. Does one side feel heavier than the other?

2. Bend both legs, putting your feet flat on the floor.

    a. Gently drop your knees to one side, noticing how far down they go.

    b. Bring them back to center and drop them once again to the same side, noticing any differences.

c. Repeat this 25 times and then rest, stretching your legs out.

d. How does your back touch the floor now?

e. Does your breathing seem any different than before?

3. Bend your legs and put your feet flat on the floor again and drop your knees toward the other side, noticing how far they go.

a. How does this side compare to the other?

b. Bring your legs back to center and rest.

c. Now imagine doing this movement in the most relaxed and fluent manner.

d. Do this in your mind ten times, and then actually drop your knees to that side.

e. Is the movement easier and fuller than before?

f. Do this movement another 20 times, paying attention to how it makes your head move.

g. When your legs drop, does your chin move toward or away from your chest?

    h.   How does this movement affect your breathing?

4. Now stretch your legs back out and rest, noticing how your back touches the floor. What differences do you notice in your breathing, neck, and head?

Stand up and walk around slowly, noticing how your body moves and feels. Many people will notice surprising differences in their movement and posture. Indeed, some people find that their backs now lie completely flat on the floor for the first time in their lives, and those with chronic pain may find the problem completely alleviated from this simple five-minute stretch.

Therapeutic Stretch Set 4 – Hochschuler Lower Back Routine

Dr Stephen Hochschuler, M.D., an orthopedic surgeon in Piano, Texas prescribes the following routine of exercises which he says you can do as many times during the day as necessary. Here are a few guidelines:

- Don't hold your breath

- Stretch slowly, with steady movements-don't bounce or jerk

- Count the duration of each exercise as "one, Mississippi, two, Mississippi," and so on

- If doing any of these exercises causes more pain, see a physician or physical therapist

Half Press Up

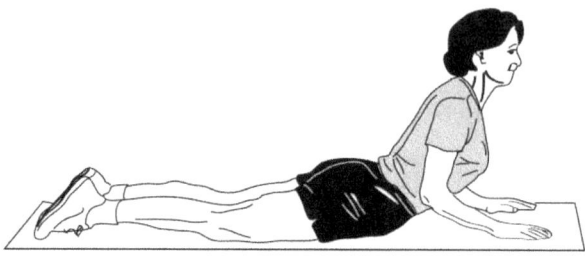

- Lie on your stomach on a mat or carpeted floor with your elbows bent and your hands on the floor by your shoulders.

- Press up slightly, straightening your arms somewhat.

- Raise your head to look straight ahead but keep it in line with your spine.

- Keep your pelvis in contact with the floor and don't tighten your lower back or arch your neck.

- The intent is not to do a push up.

- Hold for 10 seconds, and then return to the starting position.

- Repeat 5 to 10 times.

Knee Lift

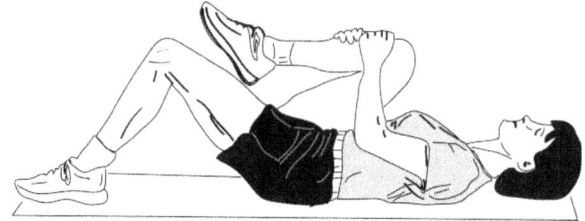

- Lie on your back with both knees bent and your feet flat on the floor.

- With your hands on your shin, lift your right knee toward your chest, being careful not to force it any closer than is comfortable.

- Hold for 10 seconds, and then return to the starting position.

- Repeat with the other leg.

Lumbar Rotation

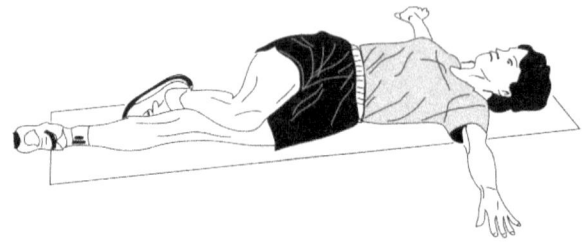

- Lie flat on your back with your arms extended to the sides, forming a T with your body.

- Raise your right leg and slowly cross it over your body, trying to touch your knee to the floor on the opposite side, but go only as far as is comfortable for you.

- Try to keep your shoulders flat against the floor.

- Hold for 10 seconds, then return to the starting position and repeat with the other leg.

- Do this 10 times with each leg.

All-Fours Arch (Cat-Cow)

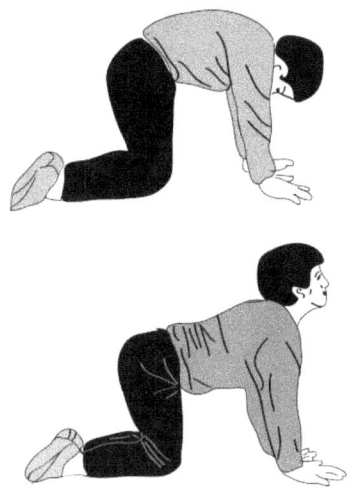

You might remember this one from before – it is also called the cat-cow position.

- Start on your hands and knees on the floor. Keep your shoulders over your hands and align your hips with your knees.

- Arch your lower back slightly and hold for 10 seconds.

- Alternate between rolling upward like a cat and arching downward, but be sure that you don't arch your neck and head along with your spine.

- Repeat up to 20 times.

Therapeutic Stretch Set 4 – Major Muscles

Piriformis Stretch

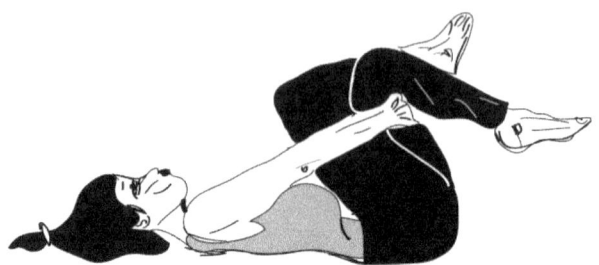

The piriformis muscle runs from the back of the thigh bone (femur) to the base of the spine. Tightness in this muscle has been linked to sacroiliac joint dysfunction and even sciatica-type pain along the sciatic nerve.

- Lie on your back and cross your legs as shown.

- Bend your knees and place both hands under the knee of the lower leg and gently pull the bottom leg toward your chest and hold both thighs closely until a stretch is felt in the buttock area.

- Hold for 30 seconds

- Repeat 1-2 times per day

Psoas Stretch

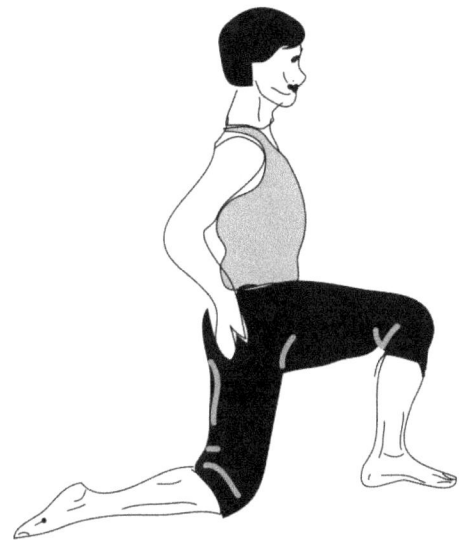

The Psoas Major muscle attaches to the front portion of the lower spine and can greatly limit low back mobility when tight. It is one of the sources of low back pain in people who have to stand for long periods.

• Take on the half kneeling position as shown.

• Rotate the leg outward and tighten the buttock muscles on the side you're stretching.

• Next, lean forward through the hip joint rather then bending your spine.

• A stretch should be felt in the front of the hip that you are kneeling on.

- Hold for 30 seconds

- Repeat 1-2 times per day

Hamstring Stretch

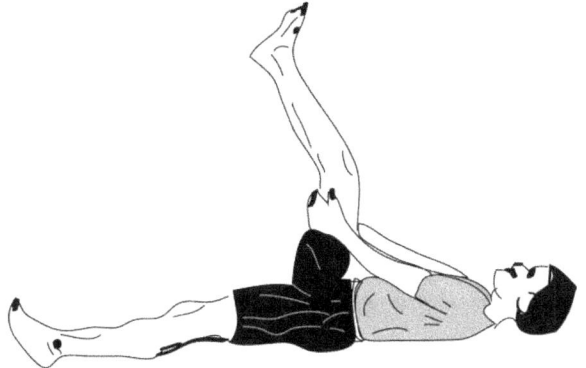

The hamstring muscles run from the back of the pelvic bone to below the back of the knee and are responsible for bending the knee and assisting the buttock muscles to extend the hip. When these muscles are tight it is nearly impossible to sit up straight. Bad sitting posture increases the risk of degenerative disc disease and neck pain as well as low back pain.

- Lie on the back and grasp the leg behind the knee with the hip flexed to 90 degrees and the knee bent as shown.

- Attempt to straighten the knee with the toes pointed back toward you.

- Hold for 30 seconds

- Repeat 1-2 times per day

Therapeutic Stretch Set 5 – Mayo Clinic

This set of stretches developed by the Mayo Clinic staff take about 15 minutes per day. It is recommended that you repeat each exercise a few times and as you get more comfortable doing it then increase the number of repetitions.

Caution: If you've ever hurt your back or have other health conditions, such as osteoporosis, consult your doctor before doing these exercises.

Knee-to-chest stretch

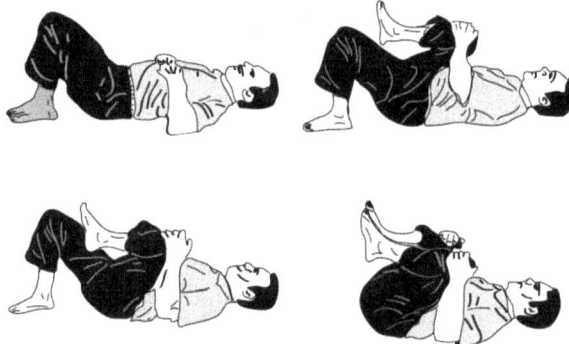

- Lie on your back with your knees bent and your feet flat on the floor.

- Using both hands, pull up one knee and press it to your chest.

- Hold for 15 to 30 seconds.

- Return to the starting position and repeat with the opposite leg.

- Return to the starting position and then repeat with both legs at the same time. Repeat each stretch two to three times — preferably once in the morning and once at night.

Lower back rotational stretch

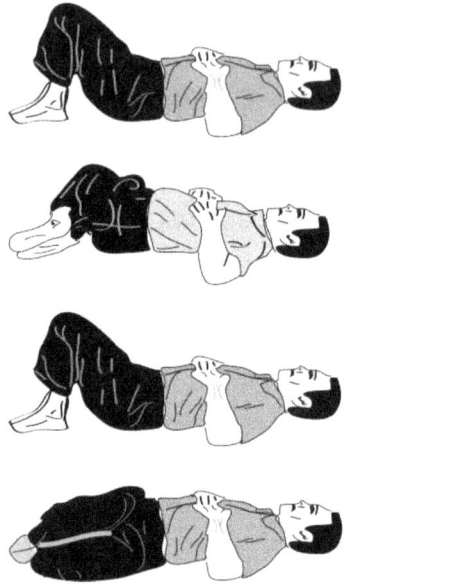

- Lie on your back with your knees bent and your feet flat on the floor.

- Keeping your shoulders firmly on the floor, roll your bent knees to one side.

- Hold for five to 10 seconds.

- Return to the starting position.

- Repeat on the opposite side.

Repeat each stretch two to three times — preferably once in the morning and once at night.

Lower back flexibility exercise

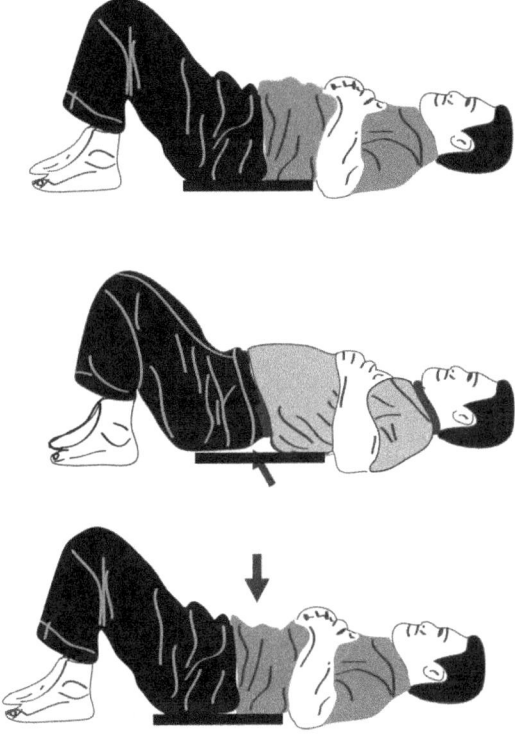

- Lie on your back with your knees bent and your feet flat on the floor.

- Arch your back so that your pubic bone feels like it's pointing toward your feet. Hold for five seconds, then relax.

- Flatten your back, pulling your bellybutton toward the floor — so that your pubic bone feels like it's pointing toward your head.

- Hold for five seconds, then relax.

- Repeat.

- Start with five repetitions each day and gradually work up to 30.

Bridge exercise

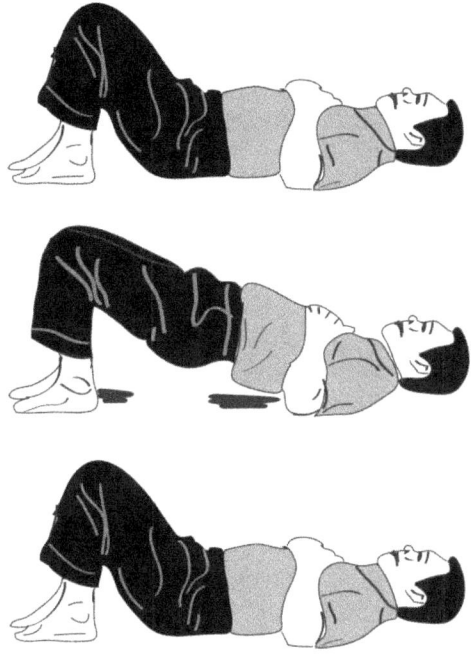

- Lie on your back with your knees bent and your feet flat on the floor.

- Keeping your shoulders and head relaxed on the floor, tighten your abdominal and gluteal (buttock) muscles.

- Then raise your hips to form a straight line from your knees to your shoulders. Try to hold the position long enough to complete three deep breaths.

- Return to the starting position.

- Repeat.

- Start with five repetitions each day and gradually work up to 30

Cat stretch

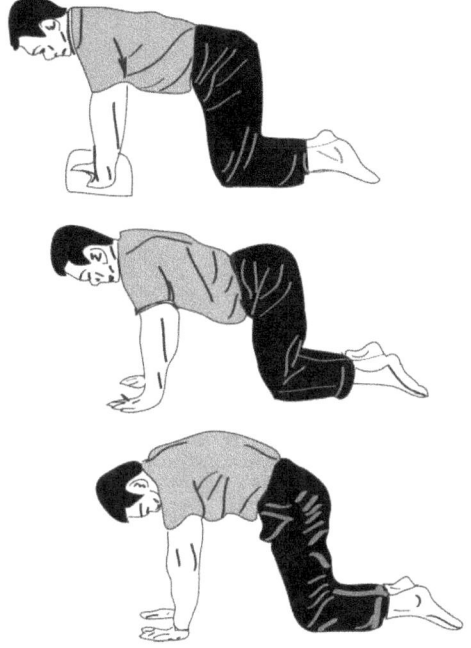

- Position yourself on your hands and knees.

- Slowly let your back and abdomen sag toward the floor.

- Then slowly arch your back, as if you're pulling your abdomen up toward the ceiling.

- Return to the starting position.

- Repeat three to five times, twice a day.

Seated lower back rotational stretch

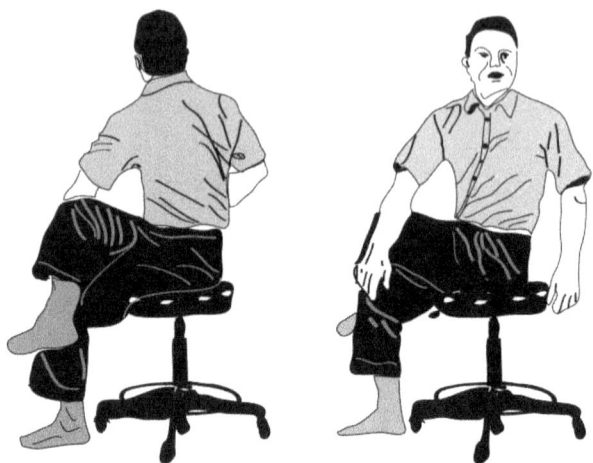

- Sit on an armless chair or a stool.

- Cross your right leg over your left leg.

- Bracing your left elbow against the outside of your right knee, twist and stretch to the side.

- Hold for 10 seconds.

- Repeat on the opposite side.

- Repeat this stretch three to five times on each side, twice a day.

Therapeutic Stretches for Neck Pain Relief

See A Doctor When ...

If you have sudden, acute neck pain, particularly after an accident or a fall, see a medical doctor as soon as possible for a diagnosis.

Movement therapies, are some of the most effective ways to change muscular patterns that can cause chronic neck and shoulder pain, says Hope Gillerman, a certified instructor of the Alexander Technique in New York City.

Other widely available posture and movement education methods include Hellerwork and Feldenkrais.

Chiropractic treatments, in which the vertebrae are adjusted so that the spine is in its normal configuration, can also effectively relieve chronic neck and shoulder pain, says **Michael D. Pedigo, D.C., a chiropractor in San Leandro, California**, and past president of the American Chiropractic Association.

Other alternative therapies that may help relieve chronic neck and shoulder pain includes acupuncture, massage therapy, and craniosacral therapy, an osteopathic technique that focuses on the muscles and bones in the head and neck area.

Therapeutic Stretches Set 1 – The RC Neck Pain Relief Routine

I have personal experience with this one. This routine works, it saved me from surgery to my neck. I learned it from Richard Convery – Author of the books Back 4 Life and My Neck's Book.

A few years ago I experienced intense pain in my neck and shoulder with excruciating headaches every day or two. A neurosurgeon told me there was no other option but to operate on my neck to release the trapped nerves.

However I learned about this stretch routine and it has cured my neck pain completely in less than 14 days - using only the stretches described below.

I have been showing this set of stretches to everyone who complains about neck and shoulder pain and to date each and every person to whom I showed it has reported that it is has helped them.

Notes:

1. The stretches are a set and you must always do all of them

2. You MUST do them at least once every day up to 3-4 times a

day if required

3. It is very important to do the stretches in the order described below.

4. Do not change the order in which you do the stretches as you will injure yourself if you do

5. Make sure that when you experience pain you stop immediately - never increase pain

6. Do all stretches slowly and smoothly - no sudden or jerking movements

Stretch 1- Neck Arch (30 seconds)

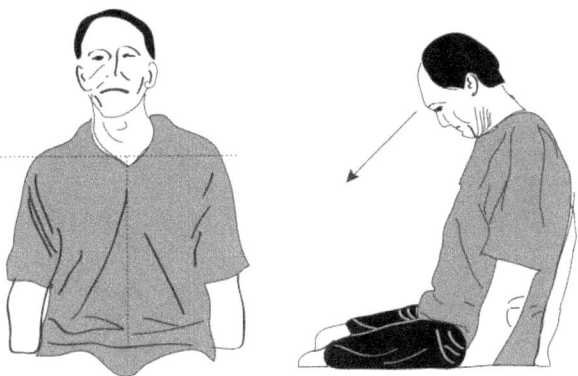

Slowly drop your chin to your chest. If you do it correctly you should:

- Feel a stretch on both sides of your neck.

- You should also feel it down the back between the shoulder blades.

- Hold for 30 seconds then move on to the next stretch

Stretch 2 - Over the Shoulder (60 seconds)

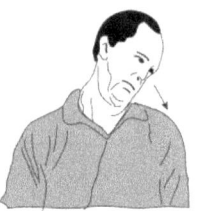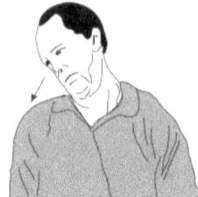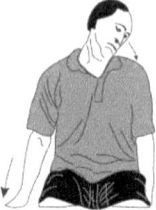

- Start in the neutral position (head square on shoulders looking forward) then slowly turn your head to the left as far as it can go without pain.

- Then very slowly while you try to look over your shoulder slowly drop your chin towards your shoulder as if you want to touch your shoulder with your chin.

- Hold for 30 seconds then do it exactly the same on the other side

- Hold for 30 seconds and then move on to the next stretch

Stretch 3 – Draw an X (60 seconds)

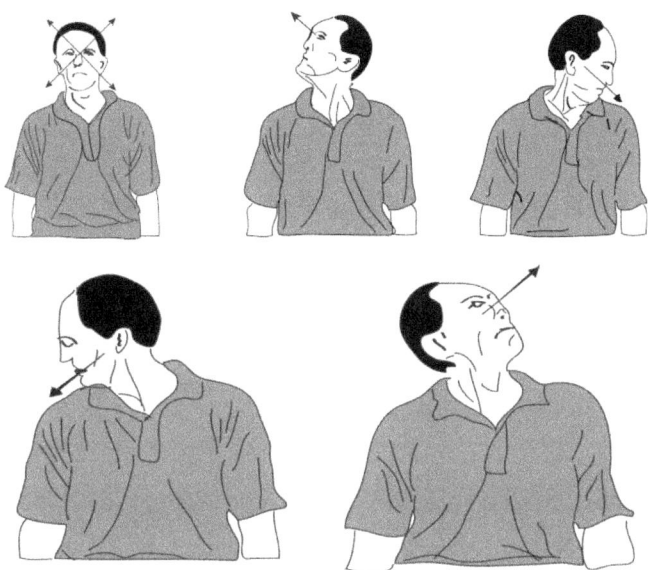

- Imagine you have a pencil on your chin and you need to draw an X on the wall in front of you at eye level.

- Start in the neutral position (head square on shoulders looking forward) very slowly drop your chin to the left shoulder and start to draw the first line upwards (from left to right) as far as your resistance points allow you.

- Slowly move your chin back to the starting pint and do it again. Repeat this 4-5 times.

- Now do on the other side and repeat if 4-5 times as well

Stretch 4- Movement at the Top (60 seconds)

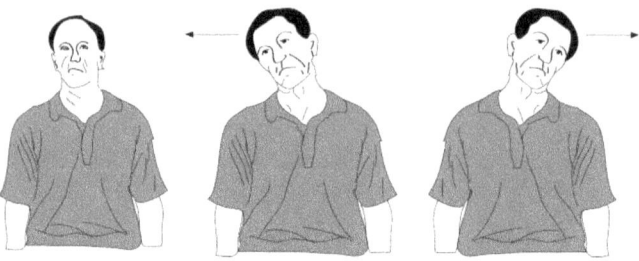

The main aim of this stretch is to restore the side-to-side movement and balance in the first and second cervical vertebrae of the neck which carries the head.

- You can achieve this movement by starting in the neutral position.

- Drop the top of your head to the right while you move your chin to the left.

- There should be very little actual movement 50 mms (2 inches). Move your head back to the center position and do it again. Repeat it 5-8 times.

- You should feel the muscles immediately below your head stretching.

- Now repeat it on the other side also 5-8 times

Stretch 5 – Pull in the Chin (60 seconds)

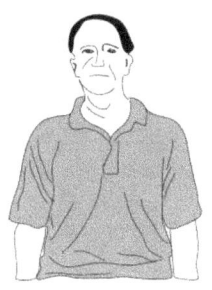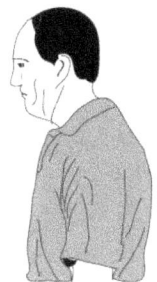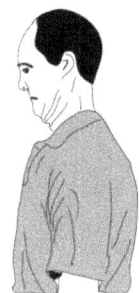

The main aim is to restore the forward and backward movement and balance in the first and second cervical vertebrae.

- Start in the neutral position

- Stretch the chin forward and then pull it back towards the shoulders.

- Repeat 5-8 times.

Stretch 6 - Look Left and Right (60 seconds)

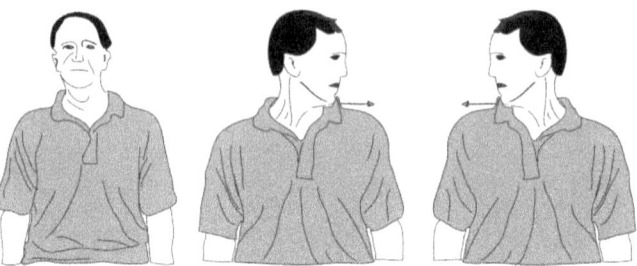

The main aim is to restore the rotation movement and balance in the vertebrae.

- Start in the neutral position

- Turn the head slowly to the side keeping your head in a vertical position. Go as far as you can without causing any pain.

- Keep it there for 30 seconds

- Now do it on the other side.

Therapeutic Stretches Set 2 – The Gillerman Neck Pain Relief Routine

Hope Gillerman says that she is not surprised that neck and shoulder pain is such a common complaint. She says modern life brings a lot of stress to our lives causing us to chronically breathe high in the chest, the neck and shoulder muscles tighten rather than being relaxed and allowing the breath to move into the abdomen.

Because your breathing is shallow, those tight, painful neck and shoulder muscles are deprived of oxygen, which causes even more tension and pain.

Gillerman provides four (4) simple steps to relieve the tension and pain:

Breathing: Learning To Exhale

"The best way to use breathing to reduce pain in your neck and shoulders-in fact, anywhere in your body-is to focus on completing the exhalation rather than assisting the inhalation," Gillerman says.

- By exhaling completely, you reduce residual carbon dioxide in your lungs, leaving room for more pain-relieving, stress-reducing oxygen.

- Also, you don't create more tension in your neck and shoulders as you forcefully try to inhale more deeply.

- *"Extending the exhale is natural,"* says Gillerman. *"It's exactly what we do when we speak."*

- In fact, a simple way to complete the exhale is by speaking very quietly and counting to 10 over and over until you have no more air left, then letting air come back in through either your mouth or your nose.

- Be careful not to stress fully push the air out as your exhale is nearing completion, says Gillerman. Just count until the exhale is naturally finished, without squeezing or forcing air out of your lungs.

- Repeat five times in a row, she recommends.

- You can do this as frequently as you like, *"especially any time your neck and shoulders feel tight,"* she says.

Release and Affirmation: Let It Go

"Breathing with a full exhalation helps release the painful tension in your neck and shoulder muscles, but it's only the first

step," says Gillerman.

- The second is to discover the exact location of the tension.

- *"You can't let go of tense muscles unless you feel the tension,"* she says.

- Place one palm on the back of your neck.

- Tighten your neck muscles by jutting your chin forward.

- Hold for 2 seconds, then return your head and chin to their normal position while focusing on the muscles you've just tightened, and lift the back of your head off your shoulders.

- *"Put your attention on the tight area (neck muscles) and then say to yourself, 'I allow my neck to be soft and free.' The muscles there will immediately become less tense,"* says Gillerman.

- Repeat this process each morning and at night before you go to bed.

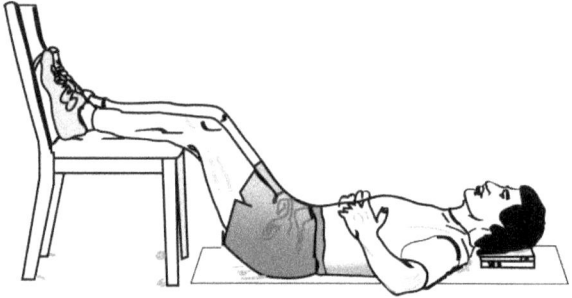

You'd think that lying flat on your back would be a great way to relax your tense neck and shoulders. Not so, says Gillerman.

- *"When you lie flat on your back, your neck arches, your chin lifts, and your forehead drops back, which is a constricting position for the neck and shoulder muscles,"* she says.

- Instead, lie on a well-carpeted floor, a rug, or an exercise mat, and put between 1 and 3 inches of support under your head (your skull, not your neck). That's about the thickness of one or two paperback books.

- *"This places the chin and the forehead in line-in other words, the chin is not higher than the forehead, which relaxes the neck and shoulders,"* Gillerman says.

- Bend your knees by resting your calves on the seat of a chair or a couch, or just put a couple of pillows under each knee.

Then bend your elbows and place your hands on your ribs. (Lying with your hands by your sides rolls your shoulders forward, making it harder to let go of shoulder tension, says Gillerman.)

- As a variation, if you have a lot of tension between your shoulder blades, lie with your arms crossed over your chest.

- *"This is a great position for letting go of tension and relieving pain,"* says Gillerman.

- She recommends lying this way for 10 to 15 minutes a day (after work is a great time), focusing your attention on your tight neck and shoulder muscles and using affirmations such as *"I allow my neck to be soft and free; I allow my shoulders and chest to be soft and wide."*

- Gillerman suggests that you imagine large shoulder pads that are wider than your shoulders to help you visualize a wide chest and shoulders.

Shoulder Shrugs: Shaking Off Tension

Shoulder shrugs are great for people with neck and shoulder pain, Gillerman says.

Lift your shoulders easily and let them flop down a couple of times.

- *"Don't push them down,"* she says.

- *"There's very little muscular effort involved."*

- She recommends doing these whenever you've been sitting for a long time.

Exercises for Strength and Support

Once we have stretched and balanced the muscles and corrected lost posture and symmetry we have to train the muscle fibers to increase strength which will help to support and shape the body.

Exercises should allow for the contraction of the abdominal and spinal muscles. Therefore an exercise routine may include stretching, swimming, walking and movement therapy to improve coordination and develop proper posture and muscle balance.

**It has been proven that proper stretching and exercise routines, when done consistently, is the most permanent cure for chronic back and neck pain.**

Remember: You always have to stretch before you do any exercises and after you have done exercises.

Static, Stability and Dynamic Exercises

Exercises for strengthening of lower back muscles are categorized as static exercises, stability exercises and dynamic exercises as described below.

Static Strength Exercises

Static exercises are strength exercises to improve the ability of your muscles to hold your body in balance, there are usually no or very little movement with these exercises. In other words you will contract a certain muscle and hold it there for a while. See the illustration below.

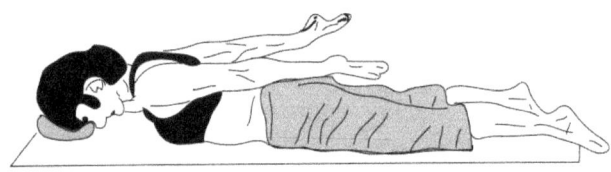

This exercise is known as the arrow or sky diver. Keep your forehead on the pillow and just raise your arms up and lengthen through the spine. Feel your shoulder blades come together gently as you raise your arms up and back with your tummy tight.

Hold for a full breath sequence (in and out) then lower and repeat 4-6 times.

Caution: Extension is not recommended for those with spinal stenosis.

Stability Exercises

Caution: Please don't start doing this type of exercises unless you can do all the static type exercises very comfortably and you have no pain whatsoever and have consulted with a doctor.

Stability exercises aim to improve the muscles to maintain the alignment of your spine in an unstable environment. With stability exercises certain equipment is required such as Swiss balls, foam rollers, wobble boards and/or other balance training equipment.

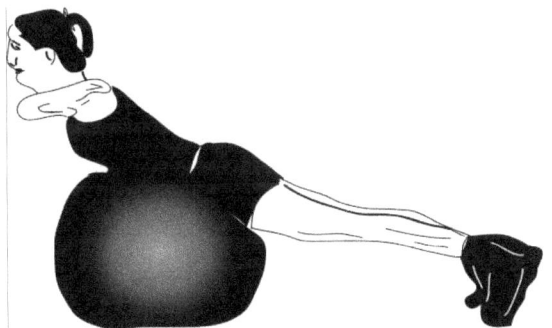

Lie face down with a stability ball under your hips and your feet against a wall for balance. Raise your upper body so that your head, shoulders, hips, knees and heels form a straight line. Hold this position for 20 to 40 seconds. The instability of the ball makes this exercise more demanding than the same exercise performed on the floor.

Dynamic Strength Exercises

Caution: Please don't start doing this type of exercises unless you can do all the static and stability type exercises very comfortably and you have no pain whatsoever and have spoken to a doctor.

Dynamic strength exercises require significant amounts of movement. In the case of lower back exercises, this involves spinal flexion, extension, rotation and/or lateral flexion. Dynamic exercises that strengthen the lower back and core include dead lifts, back extensions, side bands, Swiss ball crunches and cable waist twists. You must seek the advice from a qualified personal trainer or gym instructor to perform these exercises correctly.

You must always start by using light weights and progress slowly to avoid injury.

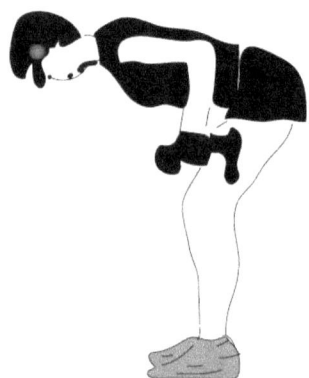

Lower Back Exercises

Lower Back Exercise Routine 1

Swimming or Watching TV

Dr Adams says that regular swimming is one of the best exercises to strengthen the muscles of your back - using a freestyle or crawl stroke with a regular scissors kick.

However if you can't swim then there is an excellent yoga pose called the half-cobra that, when done each day, is a wonderful way to strengthen your back, similar to swimming.

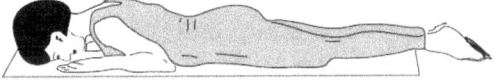

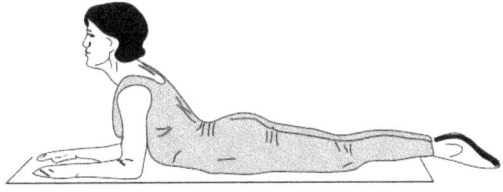

- Lie flat on your stomach on either a carpeted floor or a mat, with your leg muscles completely relaxed and your forehead resting on the floor *(a).*

- Take a deep breath as you slowly push your head and torso off the floor, keeping your hips in place, then rest on your elbows *(b),* (The way children will be on the floor when they watch TV).

- Keep your back relaxed and hold for about a minute.

- If your neck becomes sore, you can cup your chin in your hands, she says.

- Then breathe out; lower your arms, head, and chest back to the floor; and relax.

- Repeat two more times.

Dr. Adams suggests doing the half-cobra several times a day. The more you do it, the longer you can hold the stretch, as long as it is comfortable for you.

Kneeling Opposite Arm and Leg Extension

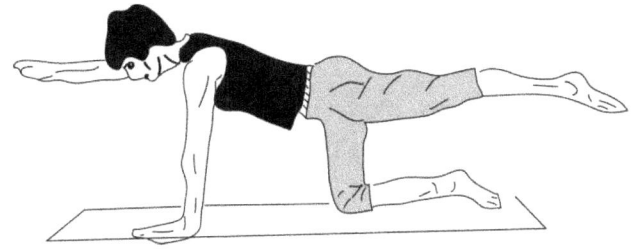

Kneel with your hands directly under your shoulders (armpits) and knees under hips.

Your back should be long and extended from the top of your head out through your tailbone. Then imagine squeezing a gem in your belly button and don't let it fall out.

Inhale as you extend one leg back raising it just parallel to the floor.

If you feel stable extend the opposite arm. Tighten the abdominal muscles as you stretch long looking out on the mat and strong through your middle.

Alternate for 6-10 repetitions on each side.

Lower Back Exercise Routine 2 – RC Lower back

Lower Back Push Down

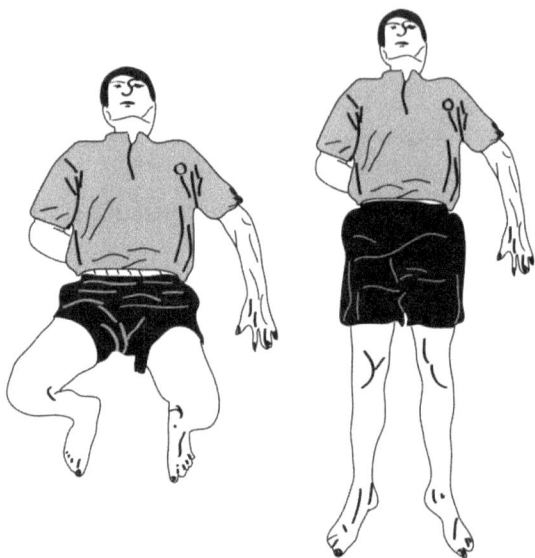

- Place your left hand palm facing down under your lower back, in the 'small' of your back, your knuckles should be directly under your spine (you may need to gently roll to the side to place your hand in position but never lift up to get your hand in).

- Take a deep breath

- Now use only the muscles of your lower back (not your stomach muscles) and only half your strength, push down and hold for 10 seconds (you will also notice your stomach muscles tighten).

- Resume normal breathing then repeat 3 times as soon as you are ready.

- Your hand is there only to gauge the power/strength of the pushdown.

- This exercise should be done every second day.

- This exercise should be alternated, in other words Mondays use the left hand, Wednesdays use the right hand etc

Extension Exercise

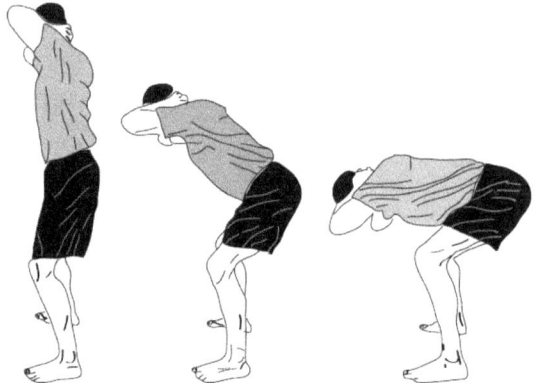

- Find a place where there is some sort of straight line on the floor.

- Stand with your feet on both sides (straddle) the line

- Your feet should be shoulder width apart, hands behind your back, knees slightly bent, back straight, pull in your tummy and then bend forward very slowly.

- Make sure that you don't waver from the line as you bend up and down.

- Build it up to the point where you can do 3 repetitions of 10 each with a 3 minute break between each repetition. In other words do it 10 times rest 3 minutes and do it again rest 3 minutes and do it again (30 in total)

The Final Exercise

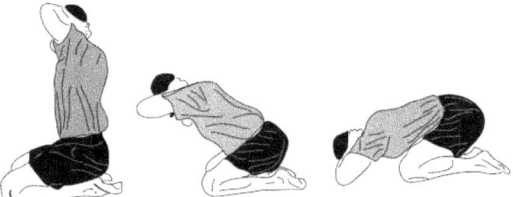

- Only attempt to do this exercise once you are comfortable doing the 3 repetitions of 10 each of the extension exercise described above.

- Kneel down sitting on your feet (as in the picture if you can, if you can't as close to your feet as possible. If it is painful to sit on your feet try putting a small pillow under your thighs).

- Hold your back straight, pull your tummy in, hands behind your head.

- Lean forward but make sure you don't fall forward, keep the balance until you reach the floor with both your elbows touching the floor at the same time.

- Just touch the floor (don't rest on your elbows) now you have to get yourself back to the starting point without losing your balance or your technique.

- Build it up to the point where you can do 3 repetitions of 10 each with a 3 minute break between each repetition. In other words do it 10 times rest 3 minutes and do it again rest 3 minutes and do it again (30 in total).

Upper Back and Shoulders Exercises

Upper Back & Shoulders Routine 1 – Tracy Teare

Back- Strengthening Exercises As Described By Tracy Teare

These exercises were developed by Roberta Lenard, owner of Lenard Fitness, a personal-training company in Somerville, Massachusetts, and Anthony Carey, owner of Function First, an exercise studio in San Diego.

Hip Bridge

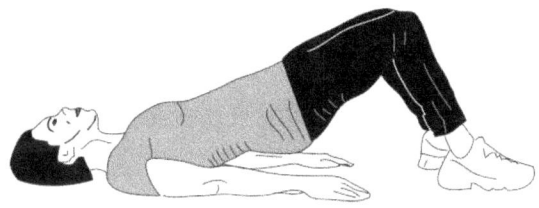

This move counteracts the effects of too much chair time, stretches the hip flexors and strengthens the muscles that stabilize the spine, including those of the lower back, the gluteals, and the large, stabilizing abdominal muscles.

- Lie on your back, feet flat and hip-width apart, arms relaxed, and knees bent. Squeeze your buttocks as you lift your hips, creating a straight line from the knees to the shoulders.

- Hold for a slow count of two, and then lower slowly.

- Over time build this up until you can do 10 to 12 repetitions.

Bird Dog

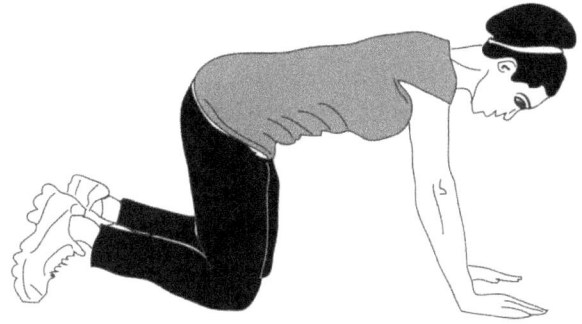

This exercise improves muscle balance and coordination, making it easier to keep the spine stable for everyday moves, such as walking, running, dancing, and carrying a child. It also tones your glutes, upper back, lower spine, and hamstrings. Tighter abs also keep the spine supported.

- Begin on all fours, knees hip-width apart and under the hips, hands flat and shoulder-width apart.

- Squeeze your abs by pulling belly toward spine.

- Keep the spine neutral, without arching the back or rotating the hips.

- Extend your right leg back and your left arm straight ahead.

- Hold for two to three seconds or as long as you can maintain.

Repeat five to six times on each side.

Side Plank

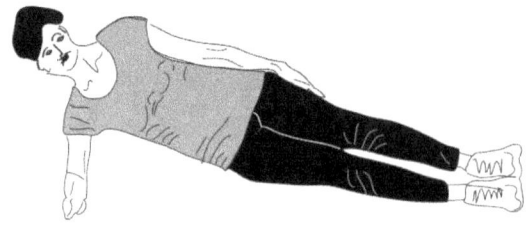

This exercise builds strength and endurance in the core. This will help keep your lower back protected and stable during activities that require movement in the hips or back.

- Lie on your right side, in a straight line from head to feet, resting on your forearm. Your elbow should be directly under your shoulder.

- With your abdominals gently contracted, lift your hips off the floor, maintaining the line.

- Keep your hips square and your neck in line with your spine. Hold 20 to 40 seconds and lower.

- Repeat two to three times, alternating sides. (If this is too challenging, start with bent knees.)

Lunge

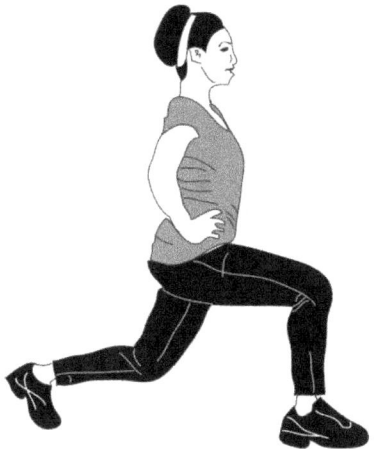

This exercise improves whole-body control, which is key to protecting the spine during walking, running, or stair-climbing. It also improves both surface and deeper stabilizing muscles along the sides, glutes, hamstrings, quads, and calves.

- With your abs gently contracted and hands on hips, take a big step forward with your right foot.

- Sink down so your right knee is at a 90-degree angle, then push back to the starting position without pausing.

- Repeat 8 to 12 times, then switch legs and repeat.

Upper Back & Shoulders Routine 2

Butterfly

- Place palms or fingers on the shoulders of their respective sides.

- Sitting up straight bring elbows together in front of the chest until a stretch is felt in the back hold for several seconds.

- Return to starting position and repeat 10 times.

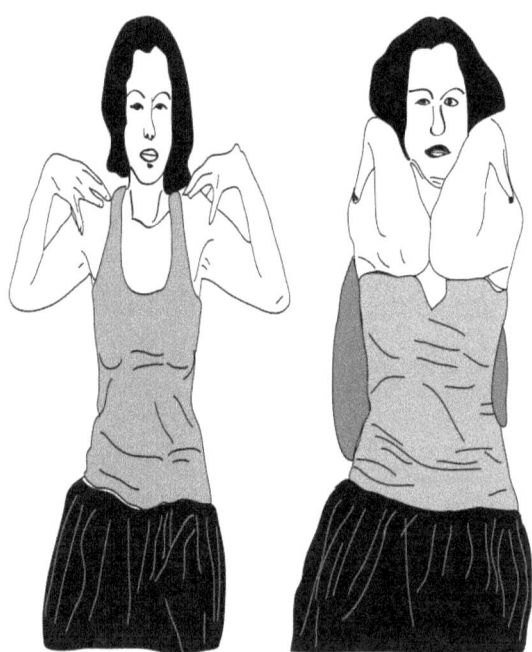

Shoulder rolls

- Sitting up straight on the edge of a chair begin rolling shoulders backwards in large circles, repeat 10 times

- Reduce the size of the circles and again repeat 10 times

- Begin in the same position as before and roll shoulders forward 10 times

- Reduce the size of circles and repeat 10 times

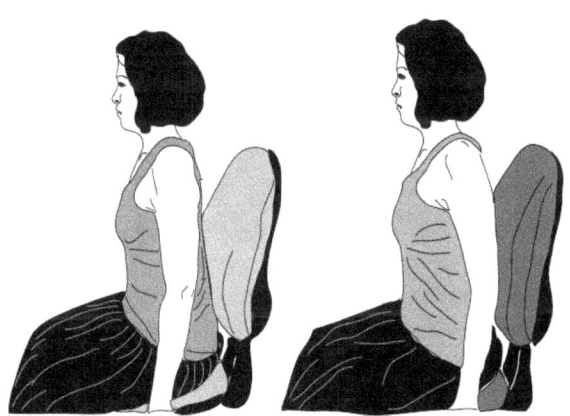

Shoulder blade squeeze

Sit on an armless chair:

- Keeping your chin tucked in and your chest high, pull your shoulder blades together

- Hold for five seconds, and then relax.

- Repeat three to five times, twice a day.

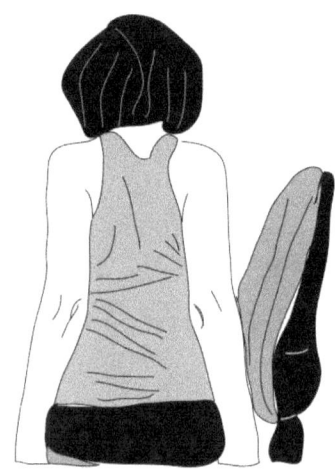

Exercises for the Neck

Resistance Back and Front

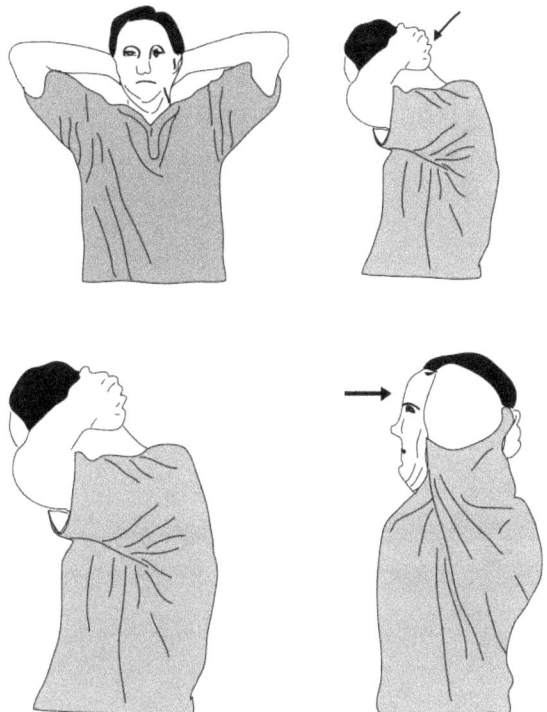

- Start with your neck in the neutral position

- Place your hands behind your head,

- Slowly increasing pressure, press your head forward gently, but slowly

- Try to touch the sternum with your chin.

- Hold for 30 seconds

- Follow on from above

- Keep hands behind your head,

- Slowly lift your head back to neutral position while your hands resist the move

- Move your head slowly back to the neutral position.

- While counting to 30 seconds

Resistance Side to Side

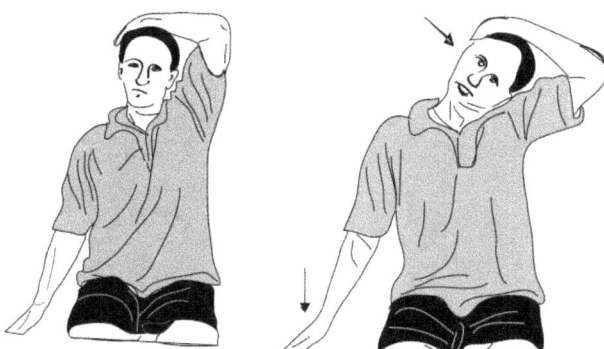

- Put your left hand over the top of your head, with your first finger just behind your right ear and your second finger just in front of your right ear.

- Extend right arm down the right hand side of your body

- Now gently push down with your right hand while at the same time, gently pull your head across to the left by a gradually increasing pressure by your left hand.

- Do these until you reach your current resistance point and hold it for 15 seconds,

Resistance Swing Left and Right

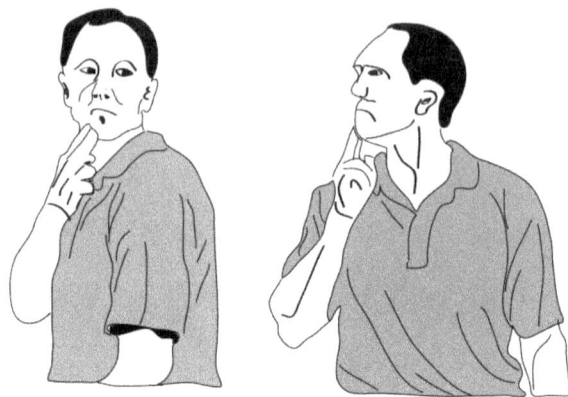

- Put your right hand fingers on the right side of your chin

- Gradually increasing pressure until you reach your current resistance point

- Hold it for 15 seconds

- Repeat it on the other side

Relief from Sciatica Pain

Irritation of the sciatic nerve can cause radiating pain in the back, and/or buttock and/or down into the leg(s). The irritation can be caused by inflammation (nueritis) or by pressure (neuralgia) on the nerve.

The normal symptoms are: discomfort, pain, burning, tingling, stabbing and aching anywhere along the path of the sciatic nerve (from the buttock, down the leg, into the foot, although the most commonly affected areas are the buttock and thigh). In severe cases, the pain may be associated with weakness. Pain can be very severe and recurrent, unless the cause is found and treated.

Neuritis/inflammation can be relieved with diet, nutrients, and herbs while neuralgia/pressure can be relieved with manipulation, stretches and exercises. Sometimes neuralgia and neuritis coincide in which case both approaches can be useful.

Any treatment regime should start by addressing the pressure on the sciatic nerve including (misalignment of lumbar spine), prolapsed (herniated) intervertebral disk, spasm of the buttock muscles (usually the piriformis), abnormal stresses on associated joints, or secondary to injuries of the foot, knee, hip, or back that alter the walking gait and put abnormal and asymmetrical strain on the muscles.

When it is decided that diet is going to be part of the treatment see the section about **Naturopathic Medicine** earlier in the book.

Acupressure can bring some quick relief:

- Lie down on your back with your legs bent, feet flat on the floor.

- Place your hands underneath your buttocks (palms down) beside the base of your spine on acupressure point B 48 in the buttocks.

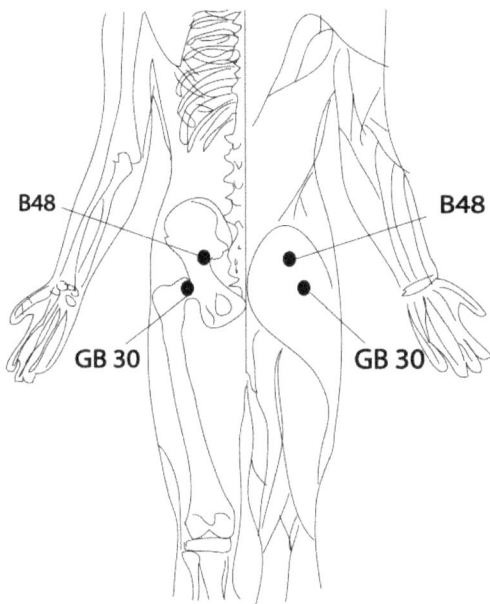

- Close your eyes and take long, deep breaths and while holding your knees together rock your knees from side to side for two minutes

- Reposition your hands for comfort and to enable different

parts of the buttocks muscles to be pressed.

- Also, try swaying your legs from side to side with your knees pulled into your abdomen and your feet off the floor.

Hamstring Stretching Exercises for Sciatica Pain Relief

Sciatica problems will benefit from a regular routine of hamstring stretching.

- When doing any type of hamstring stretches avoid bouncing, always stretch slowly and gently.

- Start with holding the hamstring stretch for 10 seconds, and gradually increase to 30 seconds.

- Remember to breathe while holding the stretch.

- Don't increase pain, always find the position that is most comfortable to perform the stretching.

- Perform hamstring stretches twice daily. (see hamstring stretches described before)

- Lie on the back, supporting the thigh behind the knee with the hand or with a towel,

- Gently and slowly straighten the knee until a stretch is felt in the back of the thigh, trying to get the bottom of the foot to face the ceiling, one leg at a time

- Hold the position initially for 10 seconds, and gradually work up to 20-30 seconds.

Apart from the acupressure and hamstring stretches discussed above you will find that the information contained in the earlier sections **Stretches for Pain Prevention and Posture** as well as **Therapeutic Stretches for Back Pain Relief** will help you overcome sciatica pain very quickly.

Relief from Scoliosis Pain

Conventional treatment of scoliosis has little if any preventative aspect available and usually includes procedures such as electro-stimulation, exercises, large cumbersome braces, and surgery (everything from spinal fusion to installing rods along the spine to prevent further bending). Some of these procedures can be very uncomfortable and even dangerous.

Alternative practitioners says scoliosis is the result of misalignments (subluxations) of the spine that cause pressure on the nerves passing between the vertebrae which makes the muscles contract more on one side, pulling the vertebrae to one side, creating the scoliosis.

According to **Tim Leasenby, D.C, of Aurora, Illinois**. there are many approaches to treating scoliosis: *"There is a method called Chiropractic Bio Physics (CBP), where we analyze the postural distortions of the spine and correct them with a combined approach of spinal manipulations and exercises to correct the specific distortions found. There is a similar biomechanical method called the Pettibon technique (named after the founder Burl Pettibon), which corrects specific distortions that often include various types of scoliosis.*

This allows us to correct the abnormal curvature of the

spine, but often the best outcome is an arrest of the progression of the curve. Even this is preferable to the more invasive mainstream procedures."

He also says that the basic aim of nearly all chiropractic techniques is to reduce the vertebral misalignments, the nerve pressure, and restore normal muscle function in order to return to more optimal spinal architecture.

Dr. Robert Blaich, D.C., of Los Angeles, California says;

"In many cases of scoliosis, there is an attempt to including the condition of one's body and lifestyle.

When you own a car, you wouldn't go 200,000 miles without getting your tires aligned. And if your tires were wearing out prematurely, you would replace the shock absorbers. With alignment, your tires will wear better. That is very similar to what we do in chiropractic as preventive maintenance for the back."

Scoliosis may also be treated with acupuncture and with biomagnets.

In addition to exercise, chiropractic, and acupuncture treatment biomagnet are placed with the positive pole of the magnets on one side of the curve and the negative pole on the other side has been reported to help balance the muscle tone and relieve or stop the progress of scoliosis.

Note: Biomagnets procedures should only be done under the guidance of a qualified practitioner.

"Whatever treatment is employed, early detection is very important," says Dr. Leasenby. *"I have started on patients as young as nine years old with good results.*

Do not wait to see if a small curve will worsen-take steps to prevent it early and the outcome is much better."

Acknowledgement of Scientists & Researchers

1. Jerome F. McAndrews D.C., a chiropractor in Claremore, Oklahoma, and national spokesperson for the American Chiropractic Association.

2. Dr Marc Darrow M.D. a board-certified physiatrist and Medical Director of the Joint Rehabilitation and Sports Medical Center, in Los Angeles, California.

3. Dr Hochschuler, M.D. an orthopedic surgeon in Plano, Texas.

4. Pamela Adams a chiropractor and yoga instructor in Larkspur, California.

5. Dr Mary Pullig Schatz, M.D., author of Back Care Basics.

6. Doug Lewis, N.D., past Chair of the Physical Medicine Department of Bastyr University, in Kenmore, Washington.

7. Dr Maoshing Ni, D.O.M.,Ph.D., L.Ac., President of Yo San University, in Marina del Rey, California.

8. Hope Gillerman, a certified instructor of the Alexander Technique.

9. Michael D. Pedigo, D.C., a chiropractor in San Leandro,

California.

10. Dr David Bresler, Ph.D., of Los Angeles, California, former Director of the U.C.L.A. Pain Center.

11. Dr Stanley W. Jacob, M.D., professor of surgery at Oregon Health Sciences University in Portland.

12. Dr Daniel C. Cherkin, PhD.

13. Dr Michael Hirt, MD, medical director of the Center for Integrative Medicine at the Encino-Tarzana Regional Medical Center in Los Angeles.

14. Dr Doug Lewis, N.D., past Chair of the Physical Medicine Department of Bastyr University, in Kenmore, Washington.

15. Julian Whitaker, M.D. director of the Whitaker Wellness Institute in Newport Beach, California.

16. Robert Blaich, D.C., of Los Angeles, California.

17. Leon Chaitow, N.D, of London, England.

18. U.S. Surgeon General C. Everett Koop, MD.

19. Melvyn Werbach, M.D., past Director of the Biofeedback Medical Clinic, in Tarzana, California.

20. Dr Eugene Kozhevnikov, M.D., O.M.D., of St. Petersburg, Russia.

21. Richard Convery, author of the books 'Back for Life' and 'My Necks Book'.

22. Dr Pamela Adams, D.C., a chiropractor and yoga instructor in Larkspur, California.

23. Dr Doug Lewis, N.D., past Chair of the Physical Medicine Department of Bastyr University, in Kenmore, Washington.

24. Dr Michael D. Pedigo, D.C, a chiropractor in San Leandro, California, and president of the American Chiropractic Association.

25. Dr Stephen Hochschuler, M.D., an orthopedic surgeon in Piano, Texas.

26. Michael D. Pedigo, D.C., a chiropractor in San Leandro, California.

27. Tim Leasenby, D.C, of Aurora, Illinois.

28. Encyclopedia of Natural Medicine Revised 2nd Edition: Michael Murray N.D. and Joseph Pizzorno N.D.

29. Alternative Cures: Bill Gottlieb.

30. Alternative Medicine: The Definitive Guide; Second Edition: Larry Trivieri, JR Editor, Introduced by Burton Goldberg.

More Books by John McArtur

Hypothyroidism
Hypothyroidism: The Hypothyroidism Solution. Hypothyroidism Natural Treatment and Hypothyroidism Diet for Under Active Or Slow Thyroid, Causing Weight Loss Problems, Fatigue, Cardiovascular Disease. John McArthur (Author), Cheri Merz (Editor)

Fibromyalgia And Chronic Fatigue
Fibromyalgia And Chronic Fatigue: A Step-By-Step Guide For Fibromyalgia Treatment And Chronic Fatigue Syndrome Treatment. Includes Fibromyalgia Diet And Chronic Fatigue Diet And Lifestyle Guidelines. John McArthur (Author), Cheri Merz (Editor)

Yeast Infection
Candida Albicans: Yeast Infection Treatment. Treat Yeast Infections With This Home Remedy. The Yeast Infection Cure. John McArthur (Author)

Heart Disease
Hypertension - High Blood Pressure: How To Lower Blood Pressure Permanently In 8 Weeks Or Less, The Hypertension Treatment, Diet and Solution. John McArthur (Author)

Cholesterol Myth: Lower Cholesterol Won't Stop Heart Disease. Healthy Cholesterol Will. Cholesterol Recipe Book & Cholesterol Diet. Lower Cholesterol Naturally Keep Cholesterol Healthy. John McArthur (Author), Cheri Merz (Editor)

Heart Disease Prevention and Reversal: How To Prevent, Cure and Reverse Heart Disease Naturally For A Healthy Heart . John McArthur (Author)

Diabetes

Diabetes Diet: Diabetes Management Options. Includes a Diabetes Diet Plan with Diabetic Meals and Natural Diabetes Food, Herbs and Supplements for Total Diabetes Control. Delicious Recipes. John McArthur (Author), Corinne Watson (Editor)

Diabetes Cooking: 93 Diabetes Recipes for Breakfast, Lunch, Dinner, Snacks and Smoothies. A Guide to Diabetes Foods to Help You Prepare Healthy Delicious ... Diabetic Meals and Natural Diabetes Food) John McArthur (Author), Corinne Watson (Editor)

Stress and Anxiety

From Stressful to Successful in 4 Easy Steps: Stress at Work? Stress in Relationship? Be Stress Free. End Stress and Anxiety. Excellent Stress Management, Stress Control and Stress Relief

Techniques. John McArthur (Author)

Anxiety and Panic Attacks: Anxiety Management. Anxiety Relief. The Natural And Drug Free Relief For Anxiety Attacks, Panic Attacks And Panic Disorder. John McArthur (Author), Cheri Merz (Editor)

Back and Neck Pain
The 15 Minute Back Pain and Neck Pain Management Program: Back Pain and Neck Pain Treatment and Relief 15 Minutes a Day No Surgery No Drugs. Effective, Quick and Lasting Back and Neck Pain Relief. John McArthur (Author)

Arthritis
Arthritis: Arthritis Relief for Osteoarthritis, Rheumatoid Arthritis, Gout, Psoriatic Arthritis, and Juvenile Arthritis. Follow The Arthritis Diet, Cure and Treatment Free Yourself From The Pain. John McArthur (Author)

Depression
How to Break the Grip of Depression: Read How Robert Declared War On Depression ... And Beat It! John McArthur (Author)

Pregnancy
Pregnancy Nutrition: Pregnancy Food. Pregnancy Recipes. Healthy Pregnancy Diet. Pregnancy Health. Pregnancy Eating and

Recipes. Nutritional Tips and 63 Delicious Recipes for Moms-to-Be. Corinne Watson (Author), John McArthur (Author)

Pregnancy and Childbirth: Expecting a Baby. Pregnancy Guide. Pregnancy What to Expect. Pregnancy Health. Pregnancy Eating and Recipes. Cheri Merz (Author), John McArthur (Author)

Allergies
Allergy Free: Fast Effective Drug-free Relief for Allergies. Allergy Diet. Allergy Treatments. Allergy Remedies. Natural Allergy Relief. John McArthur (Author), Cheri Merz (Editor)

www.ingramcontent.com/pod-product-compliance
Lightning Source LLC
Chambersburg PA
CBHW060457290526

45791CB00001B/151